Copyright © 2008 by Bramcost Publications
All rights reserved
Published in the United States of America

This Bramcost Publications edition is an unabridged republication of the rare original work first published in 1947.

www.BramcostPublications.com

ISBN 10: 1-934268-84-4
ISBN 13: 978-1-934268-84-1

Library of Congress Control Number: 2008937887

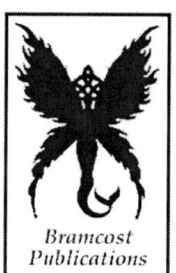

Creative HAIRSHAPING & HAIRSTYLING

YOU CAN DO

by IVAN

FEATURING:

- THE GUIDE METHOD OF HAIRSHAPING
- THE BASIC DETAILS OF HAIRSTYLING
- THE CORRECT MASS OUTLINE METHOD OF HAIRSTYLING
- HOW TO APPLY ART PRINCIPLES TO HAIRSTYLING
- HOW TO DESIGN HAIRSTYLES SO THEY WILL BE SUITABLE TO PERSONALITY, AGE, AND OCCASION
- SALON SKETCHES

THE *Author,*

through the use of *The Guide Method of Hairshaping* and *The Correct Mass Outline Method of Hairstyling* introduced in this volume, has won these trophies in important Pacific Coast Hairstyling Contests, and is the possessor of The Grand Prize Gold Trophy.

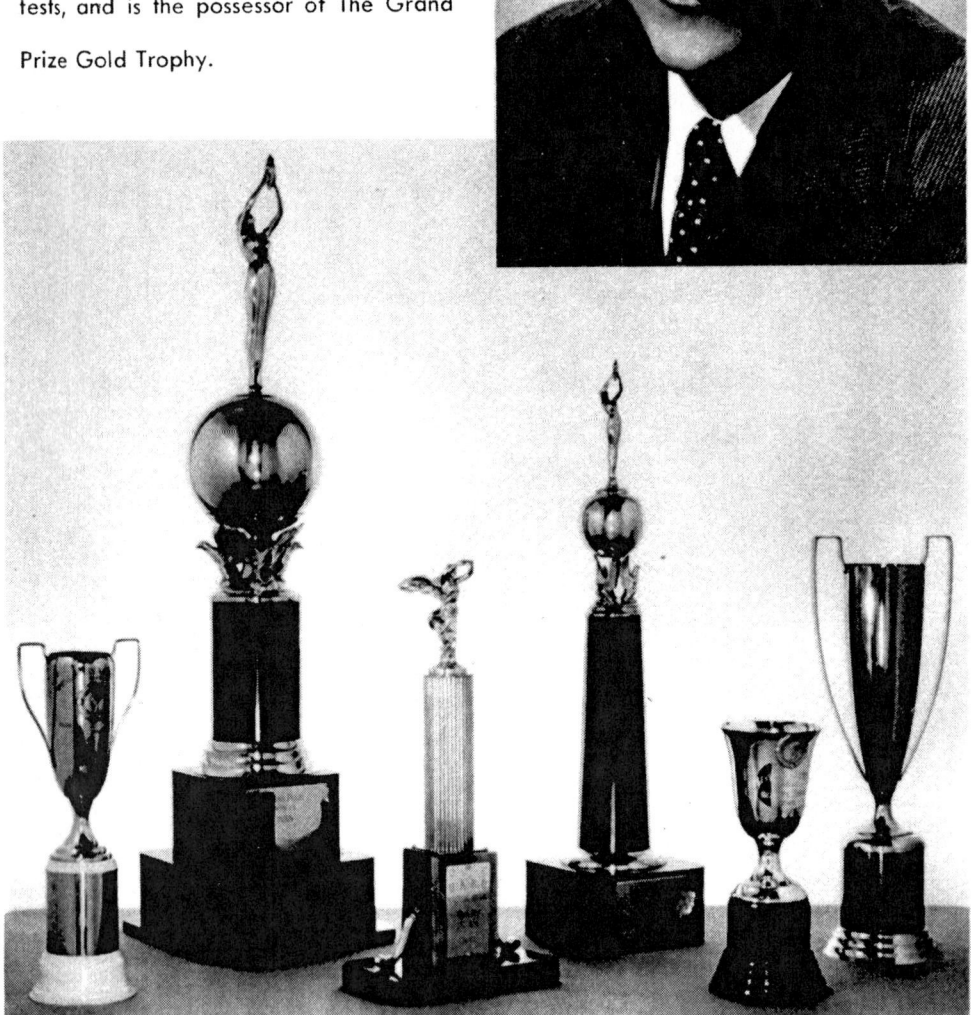

TABLE OF *Contents*

FOREWORD *by Perc Westmore* 7
INTRODUCTION 8
HISTORY 9
TERMINOLOGY 11

Book I THE GUIDE METHOD OF HAIRSHAPING

HAIRCUT LENGTHS 16
HOW TO GIVE THE SIX BASIC HAIRCUTS
    1. Shingle Haircut 21
    2. Shingle Plus Haircut 28
    3. Baby Haircut 30
    4. Middy Haircut 32
    5. Middy Plus Haircut 36
    6. Long Haircut 38
COMBINATION HAIRCUTS 40
HOW TO THIN HAIR 42

Book II THE BASIC DETAILS OF HAIRSTYLING

HAIR PARTS 44
WAVES 47
HALF-WAVES 48
CURLS 50
    How to make sculpture curls 52
ROLLS 54
POMPADOURS 62
BANGS 64
COMBING HINTS 70

TABLE OF Contents
...CONTINUED...

Book III — HOW TO APPLY ART PRINCIPLES TO HAIRSTYLING

THE VALUE OF ART IN HAIRSTYLING 72
THE CORRECT MASS OUTLINE METHOD OF HAIRSTYLING* . 73
 1. The Correct Mass Outline must have good balance . . 74
 2. From a front view, The Correct Mass Outline Method of Hairstyling teaches how to determine the most becoming hairstyle lines 76
 3. From a side view, The Correct Mass Outline Method of Hairstyling teaches how to determine the most becoming hairstyle lines 80
 4. The Correct Mass Outline Method of Hairstyling teaches how to arrange hair in order to overcome facial and head irregularities 83
 5. The Correct Mass Outline Method of Hairstyling teaches how to design the most becoming hairstyles for the five face types. 89
GENERAL ART RULES FOR HAIRSTYLING 92

Book IV — HOW TO DESIGN HAIRSTYLES SO THEY WILL BE SUITABLE TO PERSONALITY, AGE, AND OCCASION

THE HAIRSTYLE MUST BE SUITABLE TO THE PATRON'S PERSONALITY. 94
THE HAIRSTYLE MUST BE SUITABLE TO THE PATRON'S AGE . 94
 1. Hairstyles for the "Junior Miss" 95
 2. Hairstyles for Young Women 97
 3. Hairstyles for Chic Matrons 99
THE HAIRSTYLE MUST BE SUITABLE TO THE OCCASION
 1. Hairstyles for Sports 103
 2. Hairstyles for Business 105
 3. Semi-formal Hairstyles 107
 4. Formal Hairstyles 109
CONCLUSION 111
SALON SKETCHES 113

FOREWORD
by Perc Westmore

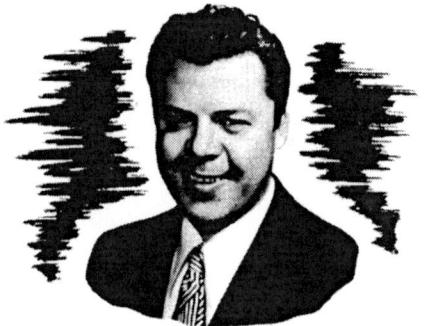

It has been said that a little knowledge is a dangerous thing. Certainly, a little knowledge on the subject of hairstyling is a very dangerous thing, for proper styling of hair is the greatest single factor in providing an illusion of perfect facial balance and beauty.

There long has been a crying need for a textbook dealing with all phases of haircutting and styling from a master craftsman with an understanding of hairstyling for face type.

Here, at last, is a comprehensive textbook, the written material and superb illustrations for which show the fine points of hairshaping and hairstyling in such a way that even a non-professional can grasp the ideas.

The author's thorough understanding of hairstyling problems is the sum and substance of the ability, the artistic and practical knowledge that have made him one of the country's outstanding artists in the hairdressing profession. This Book wins my wholehearted approval as a textbook for beauty culture schools, for practicing hairstylists the world over, and for the average woman who, from its contents, can guide her beauty steps toward the goal of successful and happy living.

Perc Westmore

Director of Make-up and Hairstyling
Warner Bros. Studios.

Introduction

HAIRCUTTING or HAIRSHAPING is defined as: the art of shaping hair in such a way that it provides a perfect foundation for the hairstyle.

HAIRSTYLING is defined as: the art of designing a hairstyle that enhances the good features, minimizes the bad features, and is suited to personality, age, and the occasion at which it will be worn.

The purpose of this volume is to present the methods and secrets that will enable you to master the art of hairshaping and hairstyling.

The author has divided this volume into four books so that the reader may learn gradually and methodically, and for this reason it is strongly urged that you fully understand each book before proceeding to the next.

History

Venus, Helen of Troy, Cleopatra, Madame de Pompadour, Marie Antoinette, Empress Josephine, and Madame Recamier were some of the famous beauties of history who have influenced and were responsible in a measure for the art of hairstyling as we know it now. During the last fifty years such famous groups of women as The Gibson Girls, Motion Picture Stars, and models coached by Powers and Conover have had a powerful effect on hairstyling.

An exhaustive study of the hairdresses throughout history, prize winning coiffures, every stunning hairstyle we see on the street or motion picture screen, will bear out the truism that our hairdresses today are variations or combinations of those which have been used in the past.

So we may avoid boring historical data, only a few examples will be given to illustrate the point that coiffures are and will continue to be modernized versions of hairdresses which have been worn since the dawn of time.

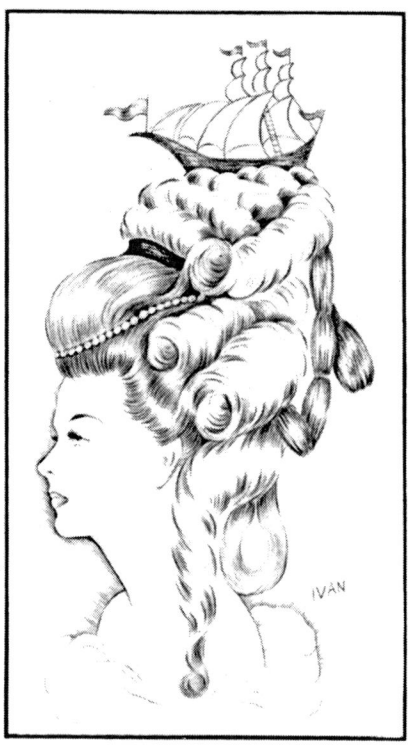

FIGURE 1. This "Ship Coiffure" was worn by English nobility about 1865. It is presented here to show how our coiffures today are influenced by hairdresses of the past. Below you will see details of three modern styles that are simple variations of the "Ship Coiffure."

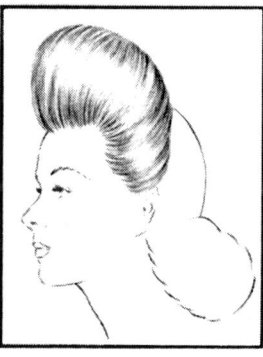

FIGURE 2. This five-inch-high pompadour has been quite popular during the last five years.

Notice how closely it resembles the pomp in the "Ship Coiffure."

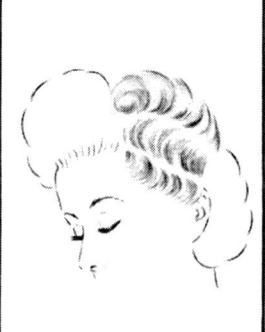

FIGURE 3. Observe the second roll above the ear in the "Ship Coiffure." By making the wave deeper and changing the angle of roll, we have our modern full wave reverse roll illustrated here.

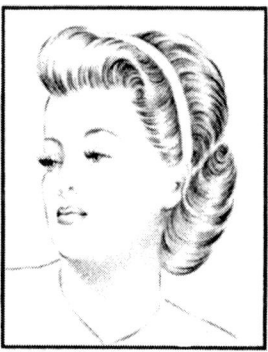

FIGURE 4. The ribbon worn in this style could very easily have been suggested by the historical coiffure above.

FIGURE 5. This pencil sketch from a fifteenth century painting, shows one of the forerunners of the pageboy hairdress.

There is also definite evidence that Persian women wore similiar pageboys twenty-seven centuries ago!

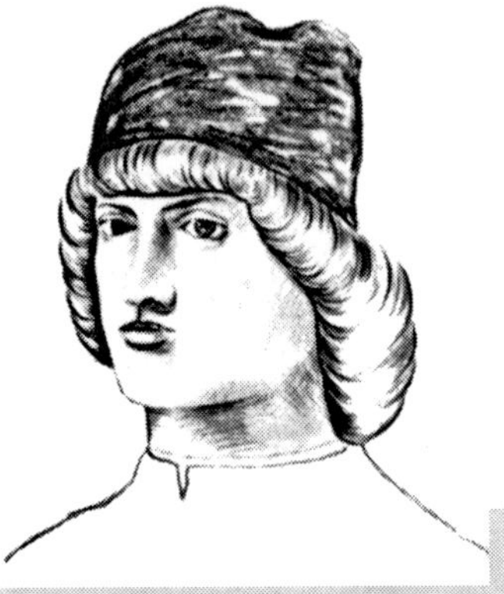

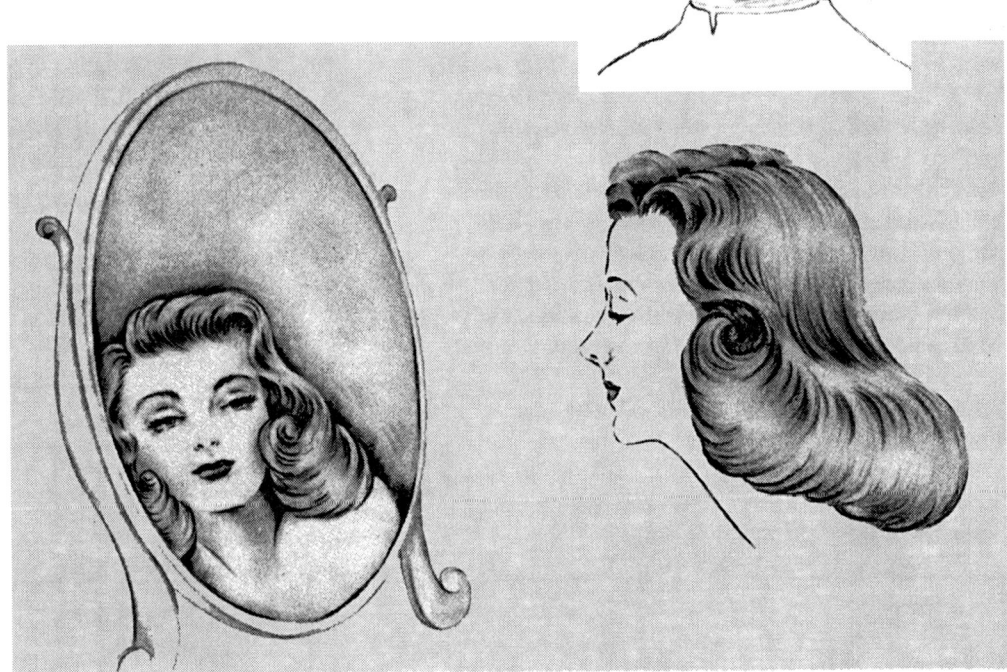

FIGURE 6. There can be no doubt that this pageboy was inspired to a marked degree by the hairdress above.

The author is of the opinion that pageboys have no place in professional hairstyling.

The sketches throughout the remainder of this Volume clearly illustrate the finest hairdressing principles which have ever been used, and will continue to be used as the foundations for the hairstyles of tomorrow. A mastery of these principles, plus imagination, will make it possible for anyone to design beautiful hairstyles.

The point of this chapter is summed up in this quotation: "An artist never creates; he merely ARRANGES AND REARRANGES."

Terminology

The dictionary defines terminology as "The technical or special terms or words used in any business, art, science or the like."

To date, no authoritative person has ever compiled and illustrated a standardized hairshaping and hairstyling terminology that has been accepted and used by the Beauty Profession. Upon analysis one can easily understand why. Even Webster would go berserk trying to keep up with all the eye-catching, business-getting words that hairdressers dream up. You can pick up any metropolitan newspaper and find at least five different beauty salons advertising the same haircut or hairstyle, but calling it by five different names!

Even our well-established hairdressers have a hard time trying to carry on a professional conversation among themselves. Reason: beauty schools and hairdressing establishments each have their own set of hairshaping and hairstyling terms. And our patrons—bless them—do not have the vaguest notion of the real meaning of the words they use when describing a haircut or hairstyle.

The Medical, Law, and Dentistry professions each have their own terminology. The Beauty Profession too, must have a standardized terminology.

HERE ARE THE ADVANTAGES OF A STANDARDIZED HAIRSHAPING AND HAIRSTYLING TERMINOLOGY:

1. *Hairstyling students* will learn quickly and advance faster if the instructors use an illustrated terminology which is easy to understand and has a definite meaning.

2. *Professional hairdressers* will increase their earning power because they will be able to converse with patrons in a language that is quickly understood by both operator and patron. Thus valuable time will be saved and more patrons can be taken in a day.

   It is suggested that you show a copy of this Volume to your patrons so they may become familiar with general haircutting and hairdressing terms.

3. *Salon owners* will benefit financially if they insist that all their operators understand the terminology and instructions in this Volume. In all shops there are some operators who have more patrons than they can take care of, and other operators who do not have enough work to keep them busy all the time. If, when the customer comes in, her regular hairstylist or haircutter is too busy to take her, only a few minutes will be needed to explain in clear, concise terms just how the patron's hair has been dressed in the past. In this way extra patrons are persuaded to try another operator instead of not having their hair done that day or going to another salon.

4. *Patrons* will benefit if they will familiarize themselves with hairshaping and hairdressing terms. Suppose a patron sees a hairdress on the screen, in a magazine, or on the street that she thinks might look well on her. If she desires to try it, she will be in a position to intelligently describe what she has in mind. In turn, her hairdresser will be able to discuss its good and bad points in such a way that the patron will readily understand. In no time at all the hairdress can be started, or forgotten as a bad suggestion.

The way it is now, the patron finds it almost impossible to explain the ideas she has in mind. This situation reminds me of a little child asking for something when he does not know the meaning of the words he is using. Everyone in the beauty business knows of daily occurrences where this happens: the patron comes into the salon and wastes fifteen or twenty minutes trying to explain how she wants her hair dressed. She waves her left hand north-by-north-west, and her right hand toward Albuquerque, and expects you to know that she wants a half-wave side reverse roll, French bangs, and a swirled back. Of course her directions are unintelligible, so she settles for the same hairdress she has been wearing for the past eleven years. Obviously, this is exasperating to both patron and operator—especially to the operator since the delay may mean there will be no lunch time that day. I know this is not an exaggerated case because I have missed a good many lunch hours simply because the patron did not have the words at her command to explain the ideas she had in mind.

If we are to have an enjoyable and more profitable profession, it is imperative that we now establish and use an easily-understood haircutting and hairstyling terminology.

Throughout this Volume there will be presented a workable terminology for the beauty profession, and where necessary, the terms will be illustrated so there can be no doubt as to their true meaning. A few terms will be defined now so the remaining Four Books of the Volume will be more easily understood.

HAIRSTYLE

A hairstyle is a hair arrangement that enhances the good features and minimizes the bad features. And in addition, it must be suited to personality, age, and the occasion at which it will be worn. STYLE, HAIRDRESS, or COIFFURE have the same meaning as HAIRSTYLE.

HAIRSTYLIST, HAIRDRESSER, OR OPERATOR

A hairstylist, hairdresser, or operator is capable of designing, shaping, and executing hairstyles. For psychological reasons, it is preferable to use the word *hairstylist* whenever possible as it seems to suggest a greater degree of skill.

FASHION

Fashion in hairstyling refers to the type of hairdress which is most popular during a particular time. For example, the pompadour was considered the fashion during the time of Madame du Barry and then again, from 1939 to 1941. Fashions usually last from one to five years, and go in cycles much the same as dress and millinery fashions.

THE FIVE AREAS OF HAIR

All the hair on the head is composed of these five areas: TOP, RIGHT SIDE, LEFT SIDE, CROWN, and NAPE. Because these five areas are constantly referred to in the instructions which are to follow, it is essential that you memorize them. The best way to learn is to practice on a model.

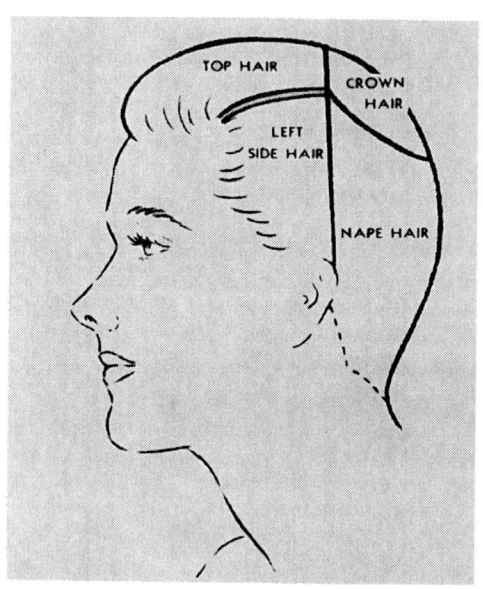

FIGURE 7. First make a part from the top of one ear over the top of the head, to the top of the other ear as illustrated by the vertical line. Next make a left side part (indicated by double line) and then make a right side part. The area which you have parted off on the top of the head is called the TOP HAIR. The hair parted off at the sides of the head is called LEFT SIDE HAIR and RIGHT SIDE HAIR.

Now make a rounded part from the end of the left side part to the end of the right side part as shown. The hair just above this rounded part is the CROWN HAIR. The hair below this rounded part is the NAPE HAIR. (NOTE: This is the modern definition of nape hair and will be used throughout this Volume because it simplifies hairshaping and hairstyling instructions.)

HAIRDRESS LINES

The line of a hairdress refers to the general direction the hair takes. If the hair is all swept up on top of the head, it is said to have an UP LINE.

If the hairdress is flat on top and the sides are combed down, it has a DOWN LINE.

Or, if the top and sides are dressed high with a low hair arrangement in back, the hairdress is said to have a COMBINATION OF HIGH AND LOW LINES.

TAPERING

This hairshaping term pertains to the cutting of the ends of the strands of hair. Properly tapered hair will vary in length and will come to a point very much the same as an artist's water color brush does. Tapering is accomplished by cutting the hair with a back and forth motion of the shears, by thinning shears, or razor.

SHAPING

Shaping means tapering the panels of hair so they will blend with the haircut guide.

HIGH FASHION

High fashion hairstyles have lines that are sleek and molded. They are generally worn by Vogue and Harper's sophisticated models when they pose for advertisements featuring expensive furs, jewelry or fine automobiles.

FAD
A fad is an unusual hair arrangement that is extremely popular for three to six months. For example, a fad might be the use of colored feathers in the hair or wearing the hair in a knot on the crown of the head. Most fads are not the product of good taste and styling, and that accounts for their brief popularity.

DETAILS
Details are specific divisions of a hairstyle such as top reverse rolls, side reverse rolls, full wave bangs, etc. When several details are combined they make a completed hairstyle.

SETTING THE HAIR
Setting the hair is the process of molding the hair into waves or curls while it is saturated with water or setting lotion.

RATTING OR TEASING
Ratting or Teasing is backcombing the hair (combing the hair toward the scalp on the underneath side) to ruffle it. Then the top layer of hair is combed smoothly over it and held in place by a tuck comb or bobby pins. This causes the hair to appear heavy and full.

Continuous ratting may cause the hair to break.

RATS
Rats are made of crepe wool, wire mesh or any other material the same color as the hair. They are placed underneath, and the hair is combed over it. Rats serve the same purpose as ratting the hair.

HOW TO MEASURE HAIR LENGTHS
FIGURE 8. A very simple and fast way to measure hair lengths without the use of rulers, is to measure the length of your index finger. In most cases the length from the tip of the finger to the first knuckle is one inch, and to the third knuckle the distance is about four inches. Halfway between second and third knuckles is approximately three inches.

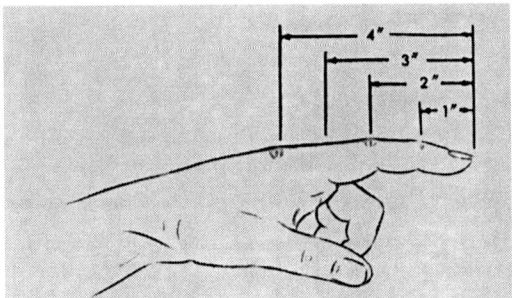

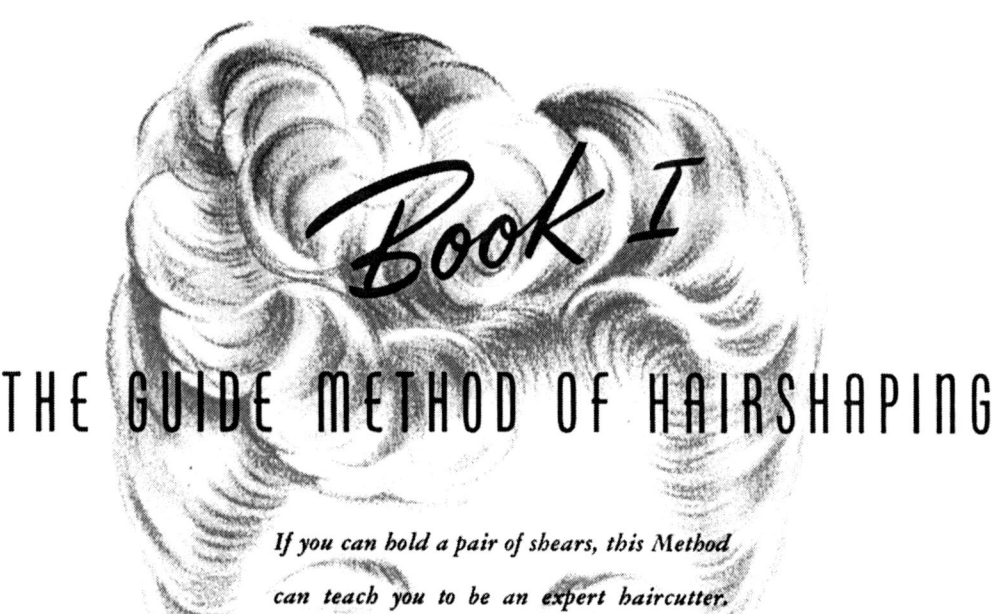

Book I
THE GUIDE METHOD OF HAIRSHAPING

If you can hold a pair of shears, this Method can teach you to be an expert haircutter.

Haircutting, or hairshaping as it is sometimes called, is the art of cutting and shaping hair so that it provides a perfect foundation for the hairstyle.

It is essential that we know how to give the proper haircut if the hairstyle is to be successful. Yet, any woman who has had occasion to visit several different beauty salons will readily agree that all beauty operators are not skilled haircutters. Since there is such a great demand for skilled haircutters, Book I will explain and illustrate a foolproof, time-tested hairshaping method.

As you study this Method of cutting hair, keep in mind the fact that the amount of tapering and shaping will vary slightly for different patrons because all heads of hair are not the same texture and thickness, and head sizes are not the same.

HAIRCUT *Lengths*

Haircut lengths have always been a mystery. We have had to use such terms as "Short," "Gamin," "Grecian," etc., to describe different haircut lengths. Unfortunately, these terms are vague and consequently patrons and beauticians very seldom agree as to how short is short hair, or how long is long hair. You may think of short hair as being three inches in length, but your patron may have an altogether different interpretation of short hair. Needless to say, this difference of opinion causes considerable confusion in all beauty shops.

To solve this problem, the author introduces the use of GUIDES for cutting these six basic haircuts: Shingle, Shingle Plus, Baby, Middy, Middy Plus, and Long. Each guide has a specific length, so all guesswork is eliminated.

Before discussing the six guides, it is absolutely *essential* that the reader thoroughly understand what is meant by the two terms LOWEST NAPE HAIR, and LOWEST CENTER NAPE HAIR.

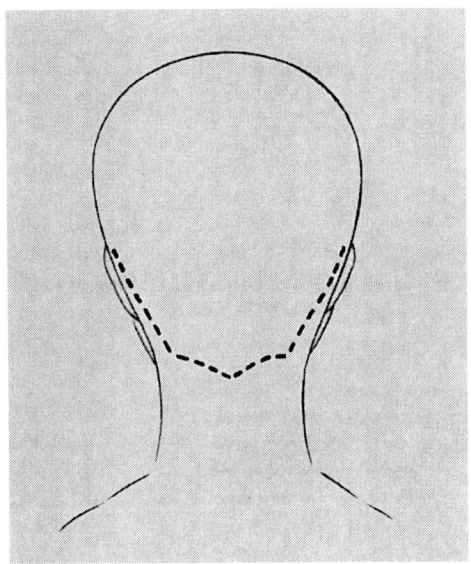
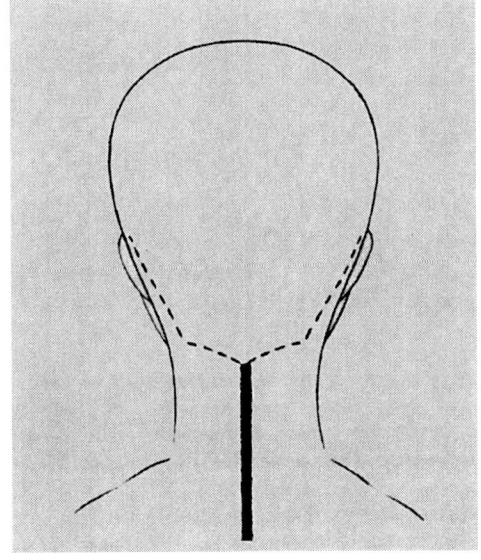

FIGURE 9. THE LOWEST NAPE HAIR refers to those *few strands of hair* that grow low on the neck at the position indicated by the dotted line.

FIGURE 10. The LOWEST CENTER NAPE HAIR is the *single strand of hair* that is located at the center of the lowest nape hair. The lowest center nape hair is indicated by the heavy vertical line above.

NOTE: There are some women whose lowest nape hair is abnormally high or low. In these isolated cases the haircutter must use his judgment to determine where the *normal* lowest nape hair should be. The dotted line in Figure 9 above illustrates the *normal* lowest nape hair.

Master Diagram SHOWING THE SIX GUIDES FOR CUTTING THE SIX BASIC HAIRCUTS...

On the following two pages, you will learn how to make the six guides illustrated in this diagram.

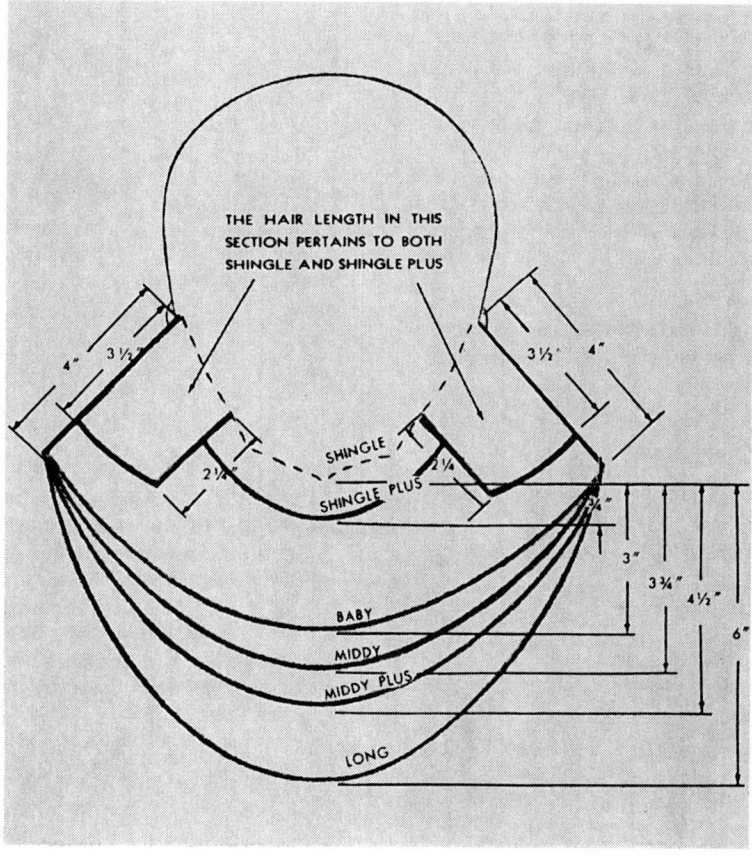

FIGURE 11 (back view)

Study and compare the different shapes and lengths of the guides.

Notice that the guides for Shingle and Shingle Plus Haircuts, as labeled in the diagram, are exactly the same behind both ears. (When giving a Shingle or Shingle Plus haircut, the guides behind the ears are cut with the right and left side hair.)

It is also important you understand that the guides for Baby, Middy, Middy Plus and Long Haircuts all converge to the same length (four inches) behind both ears.

Guides FOR CUTTING THE SIX BASIC HAIRCUTS...
(BACK VIEW)

The illustrations on these two pages show how to make the GUIDES for cutting the Six Basic Haircuts. Each guide is determined by the length you cut the *lowest center nape hair* and the *lowest nape hair*. With the exception of the Shingle guide, all measurements are made while the hair is pulled down in a fan shape as illustrated in the sketches on these two pages. Study the guides on these two pages so you can readily see the difference between them. Complete instructions for using these guides to execute the Six Basic Haircuts will be given later in Book I.

FIGURE 12. GUIDE FOR CUTTING SHINGLE HAIRCUT. The lowest center nape hair and that section of the lowest nape hair indicated by the dotted line, is feathered* close to the neck.

Notice that the lowest nape hair behind the ears is *NOT* included in this guide. Instructions for cutting the lowest nape hair behind the ears will be given later.

>*Feathered neckline* is soft and natural looking—not a harsh line as usually results when clippers are used.

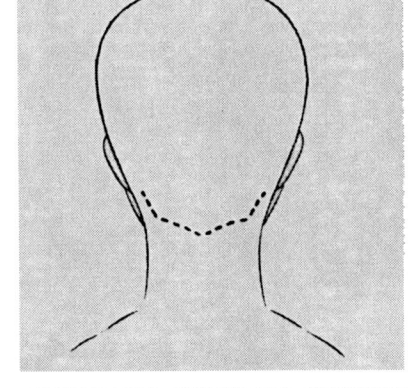

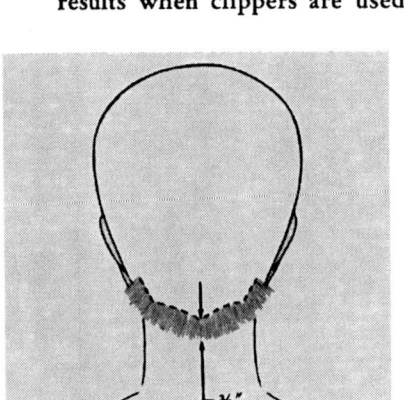

FIGURE 13. GUIDE FOR CUTTING SHINGLE PLUS HAIRCUT. The lowest center nape hair and that section of the lowest nape hair indicated by the up and down lines is cut three-quarters of an inch in length.

Notice that the lowest nape hair behind the ears is *NOT* included in this guide. Instructions for cutting the lowest nape hair behind the ears will be given later.

FIGURE 14. GUIDE FOR CUTTING BABY HAIRCUT. The lowest center nape hair is cut three inches in length. The lowest nape hair directly back of the upper part of each ear is cut four inches in length.

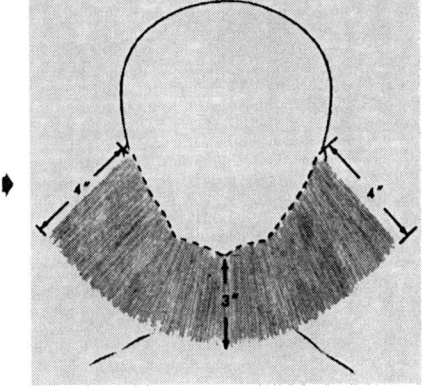

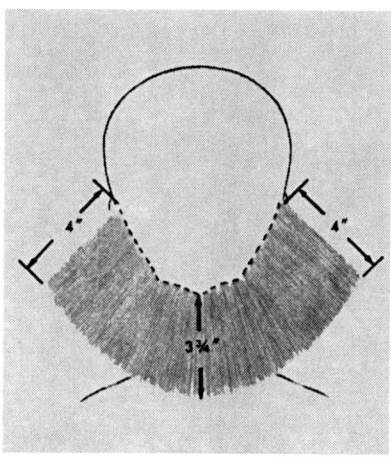

FIGURE 15. GUIDE FOR CUTTING MIDDY HAIRCUT. The lowest center nape hair is cut three and three-quarters inches in length. The lowest nape hair directly back of the upper part of each ear is cut four inches in length.

FIGURE 16. GUIDE FOR CUTTING MIDDY PLUS HAIRCUT. The lowest center nape hair is cut four and one-half inches in length. The lowest nape hair directly back of the upper part of each ear is cut four inches in length.

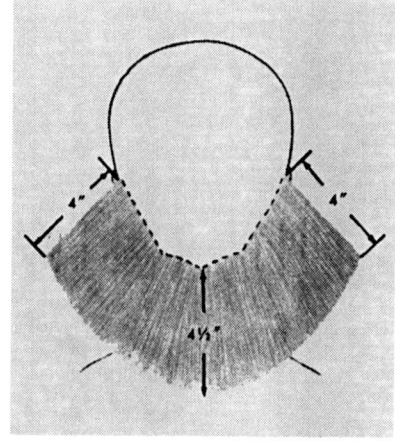

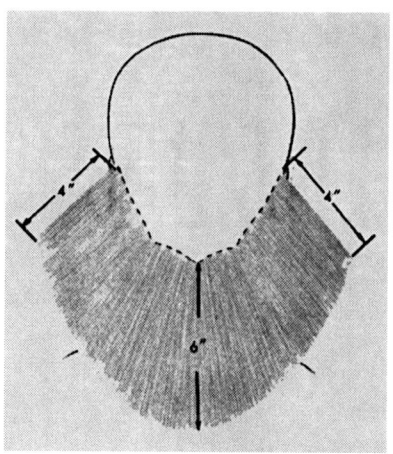

FIGURE 17. GUIDE FOR CUTTING LONG HAIRCUT. The lowest center nape hair is cut six inches in length. The lowest nape hair directly back of the upper part of each ear is cut four inches in length.

Observe in the guides for Shingle Plus, Baby, Middy, Middy Plus, and Long Haircuts, that the hair is lowest in the center back and slopes up toward the ears. This shape is particularly flattering and very much in demand.

Also note that the lowest nape hair directly back of the upper part of the ears is four inches long in the guides for Baby, Middy, Middy Plus and Long Haircuts. When giving these four haircuts, this hair must be four inches long so it will blend with the side hair and provide fullness behind the ears after the hair is dressed.

Now that you have memorized the guides, you are ready to learn how to use them to cut the Six Basic Haircuts.

HOW TO GIVE THE *Six Basic* HAIRCUTS

THE *Shingle* HAIRCUT...

The chief characteristic of the Shingle Haircut is the feathered neckline. This basic haircut is a favorite of older patrons, but can be worn by younger women.

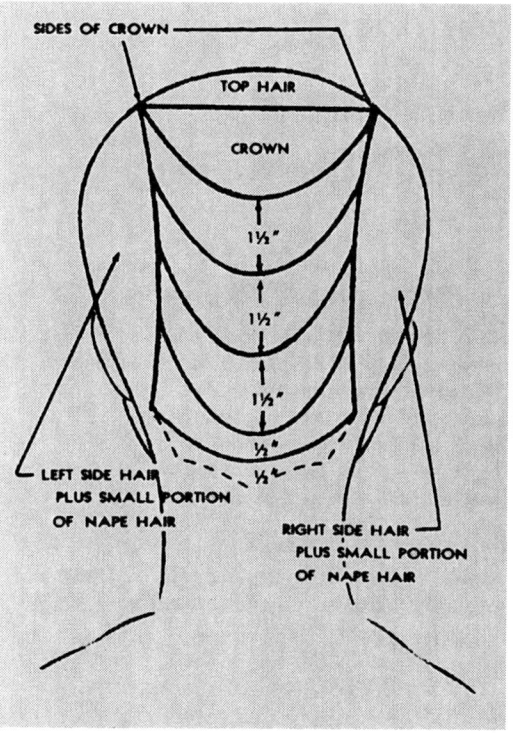

FIGURE 18. This diagram shows:

(a) The guide (indicated by the dotted line).

(b) How to part off the six panels of hair to be cut first.

As with all the Six Basic Haircuts, the back is cut first, so section off the top hair and pin it out of the way.

Next, make two parts from the sides of the crown *down* to about one-half inch behind the bottom of each ear. Observe that these two parts curve inward toward the ear lobes, and in this way small portions of nape hair are included in the left and right side hair so there will be extra fullness at the sides and behind the ears after the hair is dressed. Pin the right and left side hair plus the small portions of nape hair out of the way.

Keeping in mind the above diagram, turn to the next two pages for step-by-step instructions for cutting the back.

I. HOW TO CUT THE *Back* WHEN GIVING A SHINGLE HAIRCUT...

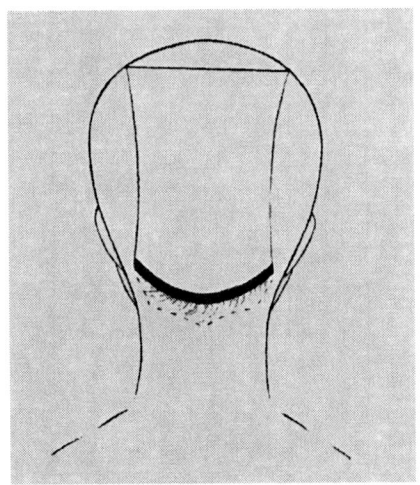

FIGURE 19. Measuring up from the lowest center nape hair, part off a panel of hair one-half inch deep as illustrated below the heavy line.

Cutting with the tips of the shears, feather the hair in this panel to blend with the three-point guide indicated by the dotted line. If the nape hair does not grow naturally to three points, the points may be cut artificially according to the dotted line guide.

Be sure to cut the neckline so it has a soft, feathered look.

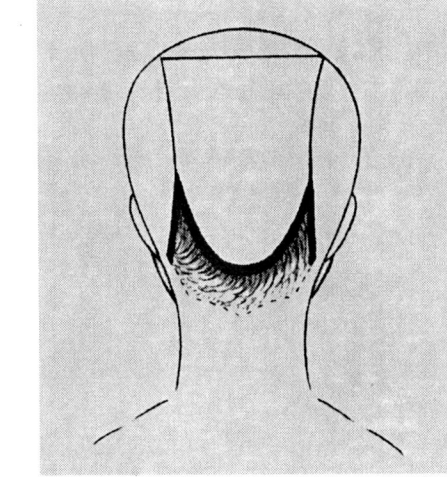

FIGURE 20. Part off another panel of hair one-half inch deep above the first panel. Before cutting this panel decide how the back is to be dressed after it is cut. If a swirl is desired be sure this and all remaining panels of hair are combed in the direction of the swirl as you cut and shape.

Care should be taken to taper all the back panels of hair well so the hair will flare into place and not have a mannish look.

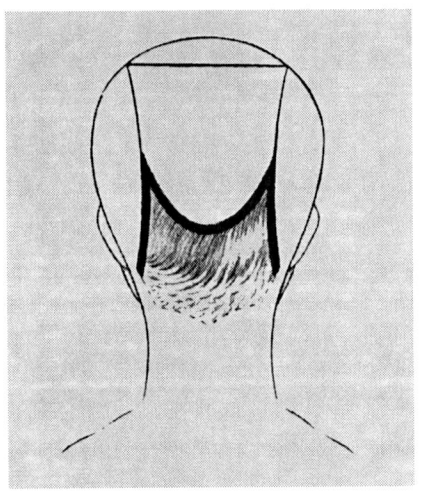

FIGURE 21. Part off a one and one-half inches deep panel of hair above the second panel. Cut and taper this hair to blend with the two panels already cut.

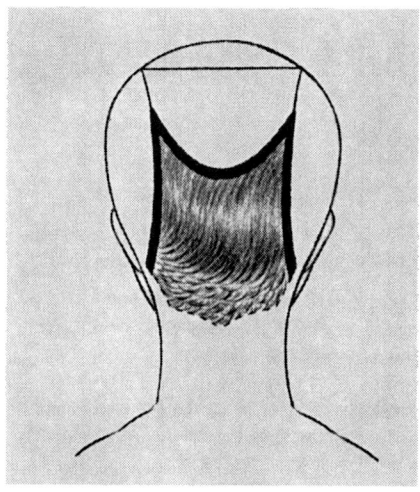

FIGURE 22. Part off another one and one-half inches deep panel of hair. Cut and taper this hair to blend with the three panels already cut.

FIGURE 23. Part off another one and one-half inches deep panel of hair. Cut and taper this hair to blend with the four panels already cut.

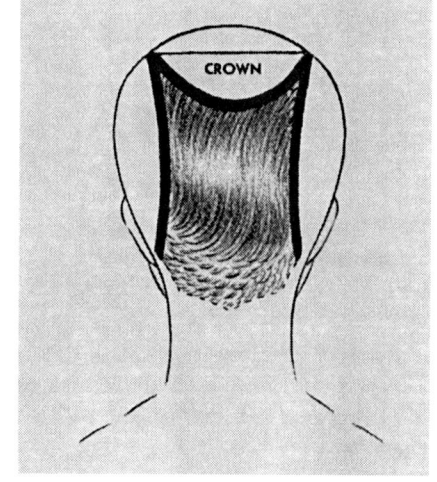

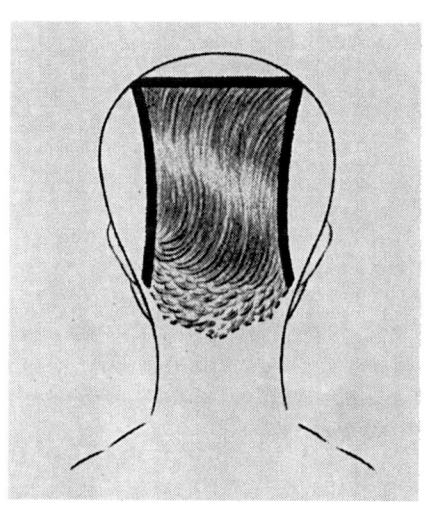

FIGURE 24. Bring down the crown hair. Cut and taper the crown hair to blend with the five panels of hair already cut.

You are now ready to cut the hair which you parted off at the sides and behind the ears.

II. HOW TO CUT THE *Sides* WHEN GIVING A SHINGLE HAIRCUT...

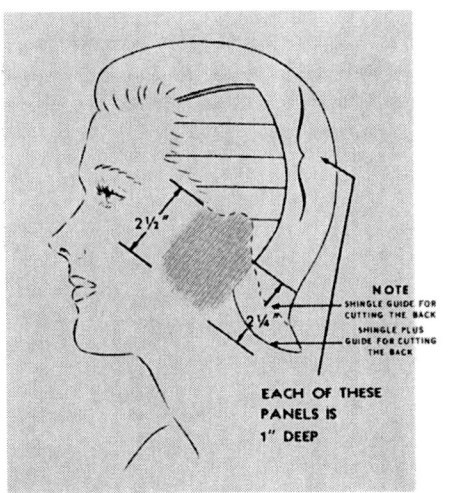

FIGURE 25. This diagram shows:

(a) The guide for cutting the left side hair plus a small portion of nape hair.

(b) How to part off the five panels of hair to be cut. (If the head is small, four panels will be used.)

The guide is made by cutting the lowest side hair, and the lowest nape hair directly behind the ears as illustrated.

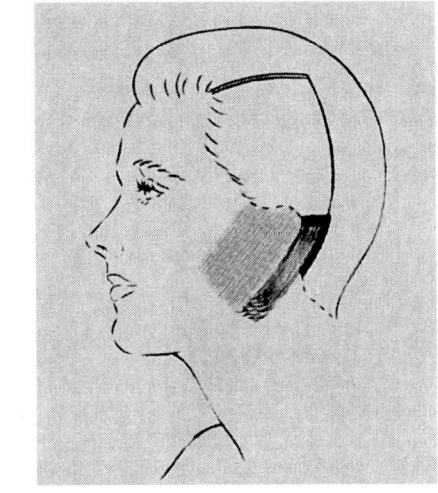

FIGURE 26. Part off a panel of nape hair as shown below the heavy lines, and cut the hair in this panel to blend with the back portion of the guide.

This small portion of nape hair behind the ears is long enough to catch in a permanent and give fullness behind the ears after the hair is curled.

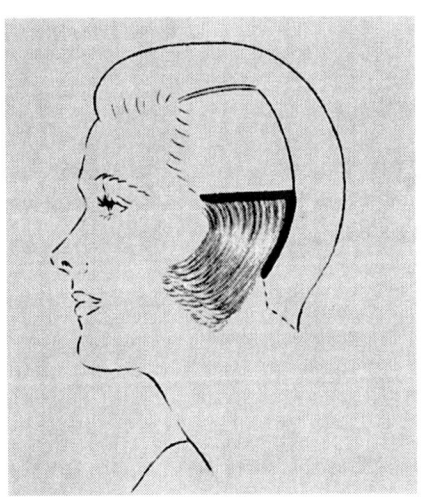

FIGURE 27. Part off a panel of hair one inch above the ear. Cut the hair in this panel to blend with the guide and the panel of hair already cut.

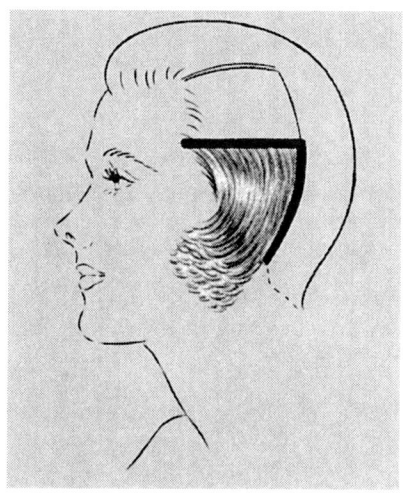

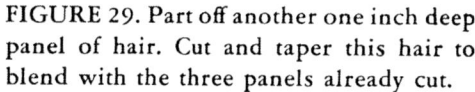 FIGURE 28. Part off another one inch deep panel of hair. Cut and taper this hair to blend with the two panels already cut.

FIGURE 29. Part off another one inch deep panel of hair. Cut and taper this hair to blend with the three panels already cut.

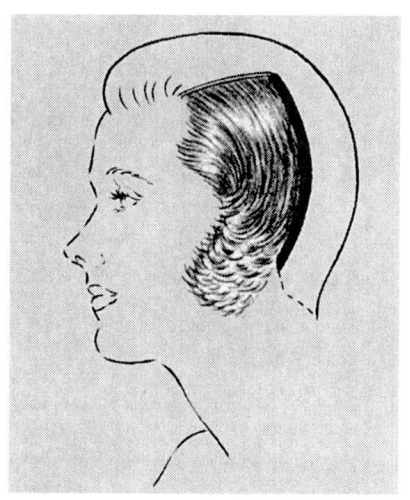

FIGURE 30. Bring down the remaining hair and cut it to blend with the four panels already cut.

Next, cut and taper the right side exactly the same as you have done the left side. As you work, it is a good idea to look in the mirror occasionally to be sure both sides balance.

Now that you have shaped the nape, crown, and sides, all that remains to be cut is the top hair.

III. HOW TO CUT THE *Top Hair*

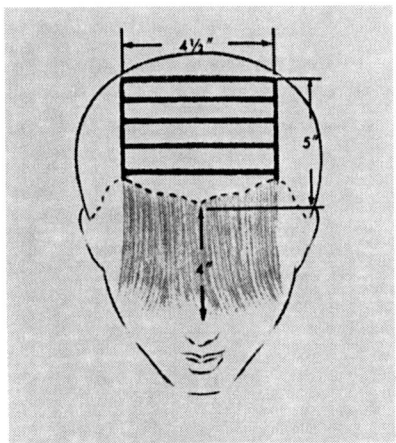

FIGURE 31. This diagram shows:

(a) The guide for cutting the top hair.

(b) How the five panels of top hair are parted off prior to cutting. (Each panel is one inch deep.)

The guide is made by cutting the few strands of top hair at the hairline, four inches in length.

NOTE: From this angle, it looks as though the top hair is wider than it is from the hairline to the crown. Actually it is not, but appears so because the head is tipped forward.

FIGURE 32. Measuring from the hairline, part off a panel of hair one inch deep. Cut and taper this hair to blend with the guide you cut in the preceding step.

It is important when cutting the top hair to comb each panel of hair forward, and stand in front of the patron while shaping. This causes the top hair to blend perfectly with the rest of the haircut, and also makes it possible for the patron to change her part anytime she desires.

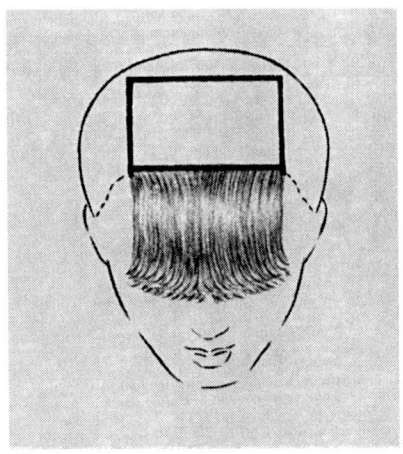

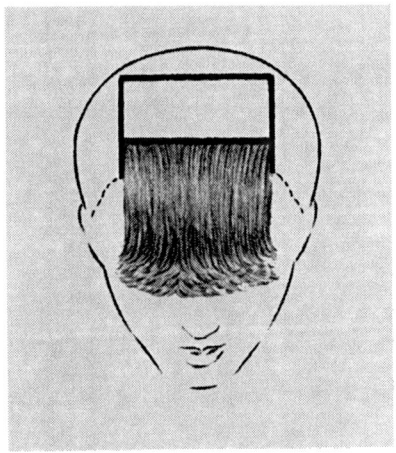

FIGURE 33. Part off another one inch deep panel of hair. Cut and taper this hair to blend with the first panel already cut.

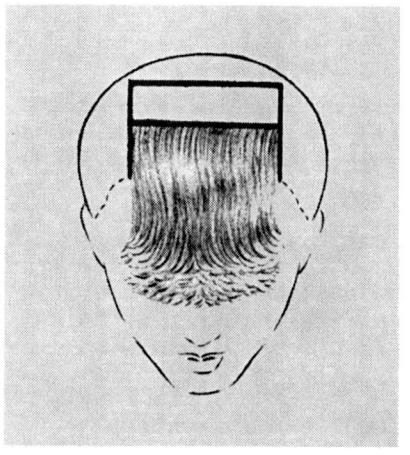

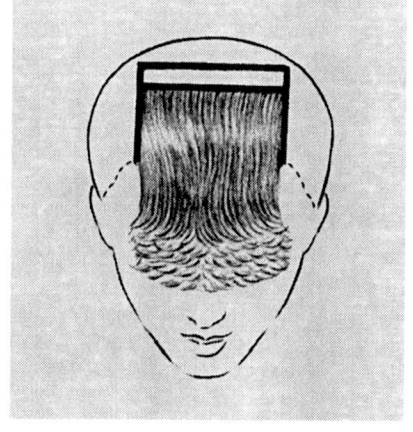

FIGURE 34. Part off another one inch deep panel of hair. Cut and taper this hair to blend with the two panels already cut.

FIGURE 35. Part off another one inch deep panel of hair. Cut and taper this hair to blend with the three panels already cut.

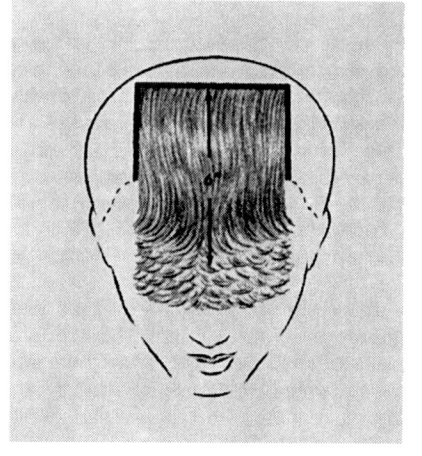

FIGURE 36. Bring down the remaining top hair and cut it to blend with the four panels already cut.

Notice that the top hair varies in length from four inches at the hairline to six inches in back, and that there are no definite step-offs because the hair has been properly shaped.

REMEMBER THIS: *The instructions for cutting the top hair on these two pages apply to the cutting of these five Basic Haircuts: Shingle, Shingle Plus, Middy, Middy Plus, and Long. The only Basic Haircut exception is the Baby Haircut. When giving a Baby Haircut ALL the top hair is cut three inches in length as explained later.*

THE *Shingle Plus* HAIRCUT...

The Shingle Plus Haircut is just like the Shingle Haircut except the guide is three-quarters of an inch longer than the feathered three point neckline of the Shingle Haircut, and the hair in the panel illustrated in Figure 38, is left long enough to blend with the Shingle Plus guide.

A word of caution. If the nape hair near the neckline is straight and grows in a downward direction, the Shingle Plus Haircut will not be practical because the lowest panel of hair would be too short to permanent wave, and would stand out from the head in an unbecoming way. However, this is an ideal haircut for women who have naturally curly hair or for those few who have nape hair that grows in an upward direction at the neckline.

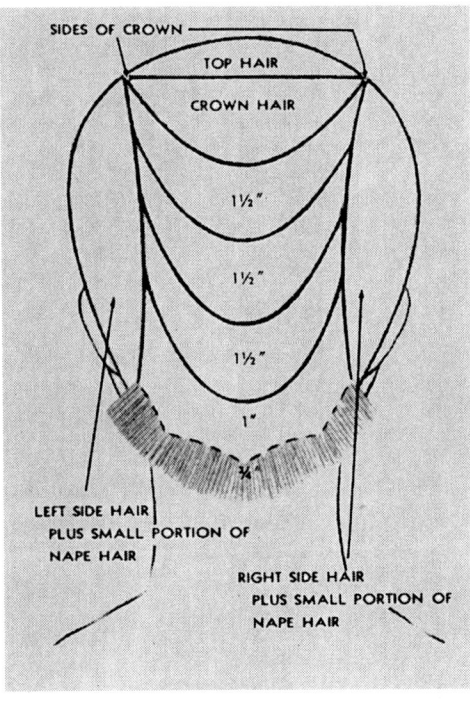

FIGURE 37. This diagram shows:

(a) The guide (illustrated by the up and down lines.)

(b) How to part off the five panels of hair to be cut first.

First, section off the top hair and pin it out of the way. (The same as you did when giving the Shingle Haircut).

Next, make two parts from the sides of the crown down to about one-half inch behind the bottom of each ear. Observe that these two parts *curve inward* toward the ear lobes, and in this way small portions of the nape hair are included with the left and right side hair so there will be extra fullness at the sides and behind the ears after the hair is dressed.

Pin the right and left side hair plus the small portions of nape hair out of the way. (This procedure is the same as you followed when giving the Shingle Haircut.)

The guide is made by cutting the lowest center nape hair and that section of the lowest nape hair indicated by the up and down lines, three-quarters of an inch in length.

Notice in the diagram above that the panels of hair are parted off the same as you did when giving a Shingle Haircut, except the lowest panel is one inch deep.

Keeping in mind the above diagram, study the next page for instructions for cutting the back.

I. HOW TO CUT THE *Back* WHEN GIVING A SHINGLE PLUS HAIRCUT...

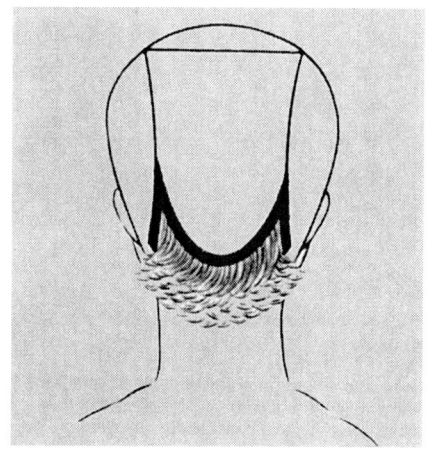

FIGURE 38. Measuring up from the lowest center nape hair, part off a panel of hair one inch deep as illustrated below the heavy lines.

Cut and taper the hair in this panel to blend with the guide.

Now continue cutting the remaining four panels of hair exactly the same as you did on pages 22 and 23 when you gave a Shingle Haircut.

You are now ready to cut and shape the hair which you parted off at the sides and behind the ears.

II. HOW TO CUT THE *Sides* WHEN GIVING A SHINGLE PLUS HAIRCUT...

FIGURE 39. This diagram shows:

(a) The guide for cutting the left side hair plus a small portion of the nape hair.

(b) How to part off the five panels of hair to be cut. (The same as you did when giving the Shingle Haircut.)

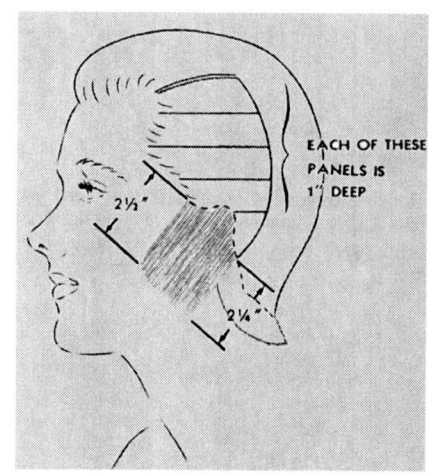

The guide is made by cutting the lowest side hair and the lowest nape hair directly behind the ears as illustrated. (The same as you did when giving the Shingle Haircut.)

The side view of the guide used for cutting the back is also indicated in this diagram.

Since the instructions for cutting the sides are *exactly the same* as you followed when giving the Shingle Haircut, they will not be repeated here. Turn to pages 24 and 25, and cut the left and right sides according to the instructions on those two pages.

III. HOW TO CUT THE *Top Hair* WHEN GIVING A SHINGLE PLUS HAIRCUT...

Turn to pages 26 and 27, and cut the top hair exactly as explained on those two pages.

THE *Baby* HAIRCUT...

The chief characteristic of the Baby Haircut is that all the hair on the head is cut three inches in length EXCEPT the hair around the ears. The Baby Haircut is recommended *only* for those very few women who have thick hair and desire to wear a loose, casual hairdress.

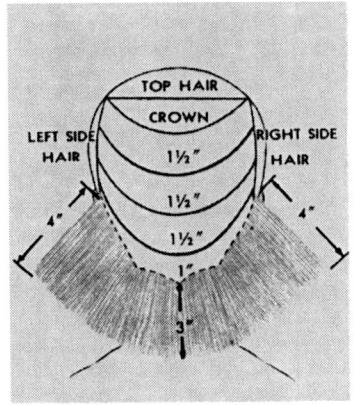

FIGURE 40. This diagram shows:

   (a) The guide.

   (b) How to part off the five panels of nape and crown hair to be cut.

First, section off the top hair and pin it out of the way. (The same as you did when giving the Shingle and Shingle Plus Haircuts.)

Next, make two crown-to-ear parts and pin the left and right side hair out of the way.

> NOTE: The two crown-to-ear parts are straight up and down (See page 46, Figure 70 for definition of a crown-to-ear part), but appear to have a slight curve because we are seeing them from a back view.

The guide is made by cutting the lowest center nape hair three inches in length. The lowest nape hair directly behind the upper part of the ears is cut four inches in length in order to provide fullness behind the ears after the hair is dressed.

I. HOW TO CUT THE *Nape* AND *Crown Hair* WHEN GIVING A BABY HAIRCUT...

FIGURE 41. Measuring up from the lowest center nape hair, part off a panel of hair one inch deep as illustrated below the heavy line. Cut and taper the hair in this panel to blend with the guide.

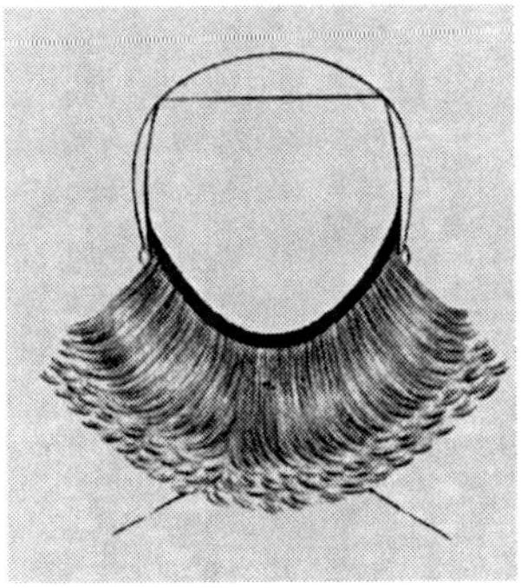

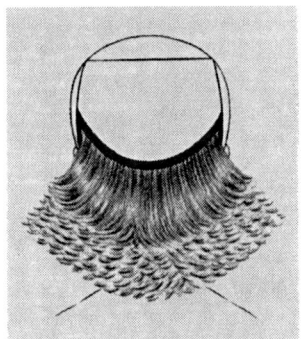

FIGURE 42. Part off a panel of nape hair one and one-half inches deep above the first panel.

Cut and taper this panel of hair to blend with the first panel of hair already cut.

Cut and taper all the nape and crown hair in the remaining three panels three inches in length. Make measurements with forefinger while holding the hair straight out from the head.

You are now ready to cut the left and right side hair.

II. HOW TO CUT THE *Sides* WHEN GIVING A BABY HAIRCUT...

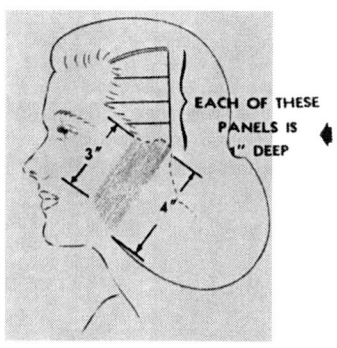

FIGURE 43. This diagram shows:
  (a) The guide for cutting the left side hair.
  (b) How to part off the four panels of side hair to be cut. (If the head is small, three panels will be used.)

The guide is made by cutting the lowest side hair according to the dimensions given in the illustration. From a side view, notice how the length of the guide for cutting the side hair blends into one continuous line with the length and shape of the Baby Haircut in back.

FIGURE 44. Part off a panel of side hair one inch above the ear.

Cut and taper the hair in this panel to blend with the guide as illustrated.

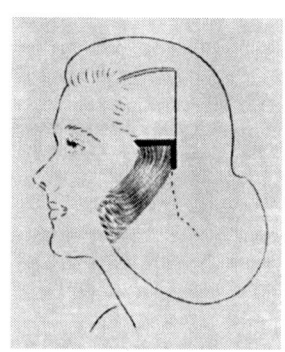

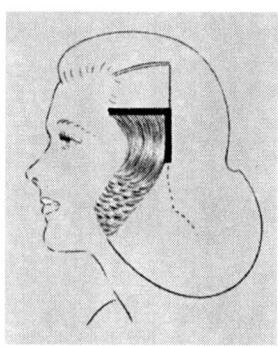

FIGURE 45. Part off another one inch deep panel of side hair and cut this hair to blend with the first panel of hair already cut.

Cut and taper all the hair in the remaining two panels of side hair three inches in length. Make measurements while holding the hair straight out from the head.

Next, cut the right side hair exactly the same as you have done the left side. Now that you have cut the nape, crown, and sides, all that remains to be cut is the top hair.

III. HOW TO CUT THE *Top Hair* WHEN GIVING A BABY HAIRCUT...

FIGURE 46. This diagram shows:
  (a) How to part off the five panels of top hair prior to cutting. (Each panel is one inch deep.)

Cut and taper the hair in each of these five panels to a three inch length. Make measurements while holding the hair straight out from the head.

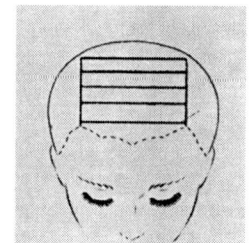

THE *Middy* HAIRCUT...

The author introduced the Middy Haircut to the Hairdressing Profession at the Los Angeles Trade Show. It is called Middy because it is neither too short nor too long—it is the ideal haircut for almost all American women, and is adaptable to dozens of different hairstyles. Beauty Shops all over the country have adopted the Middy Haircut, and have featured it under no less than fifty different names. For this reason, it is safe to say that the Middy Haircut is the most popular haircut of the century.

FIGURE 47. This diagram shows:

(a) The guide.

(b) How to part off the five panels of nape and crown hair to be cut. (The same as you did when giving the Baby Haircut.)

First, section off the top hair and pin it out of the way. (The same as you did when giving the Shingle, Shingle Plus and Baby Haircuts.)

Next, make two crown-to-ear parts, and pin the left and right side hair out of the way. (The same as you did when giving the Baby Haircut.)

The guide is made by cutting the lowest center nape hair three and three-quarters inches in length. The lowest nape hair directly behind the upper part of the ears is cut four inches in length.

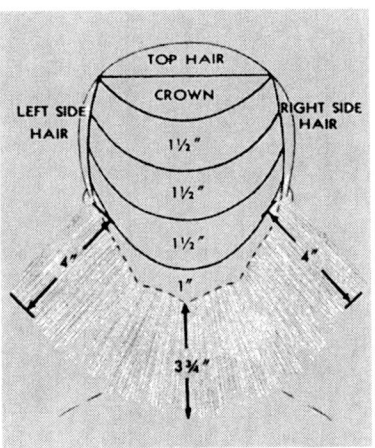

I. HOW TO CUT THE *Nape* AND *Crown Hair* WHEN GIVING A MIDDY HAIRCUT...

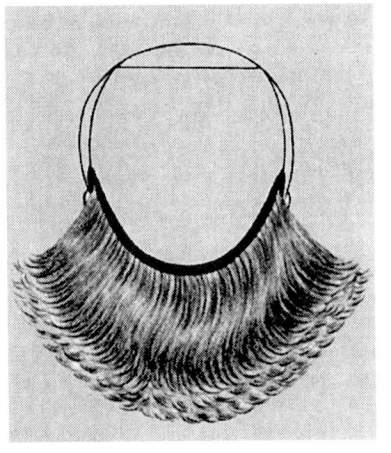

FIGURE 48. Measuring up from the lowest center nape hair, part off a panel of hair one inch deep as illustrated below the heavy line.

Cut and taper this hair to blend with the guide.

FIGURE 49. Part off a panel of hair one and one-half inches deep.

Cut and taper this hair to blend with the first panel already cut.

This illustration shows the hair being cut with a razor, but shears may be used if you prefer.

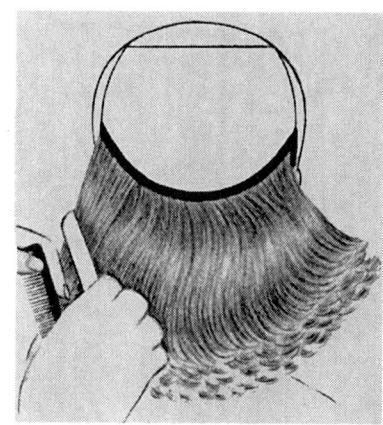

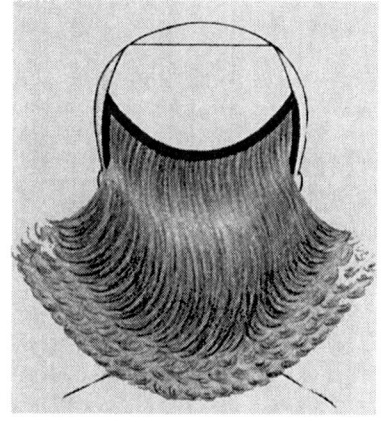

FIGURE 50. Part off another panel of hair one and one-half inches deep.

Cut and taper this hair to blend with the two panels already cut.

FIGURE 51. Part off another panel of hair one and one-half inches deep.

Cut and taper this hair to blend with the three panels already cut.

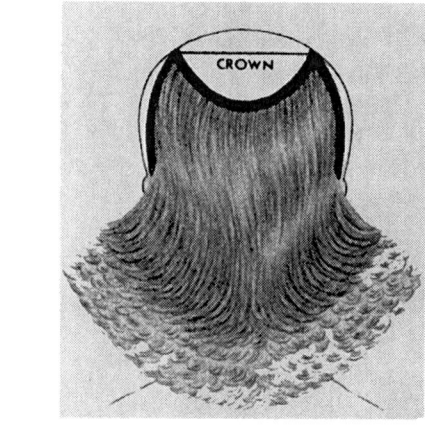

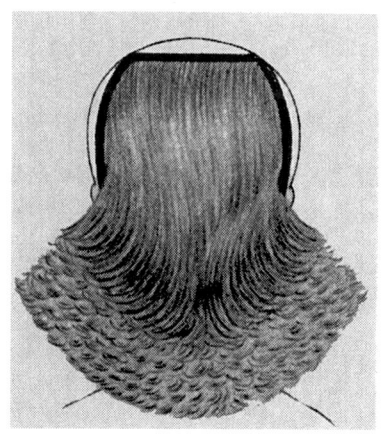

FIGURE 52. Bring down the crown hair and cut it to blend with the four panels of hair already cut.

You are now ready to cut the left and right side hair.

II. HOW TO CUT THE *Sides* WHEN GIVING A MIDDY HAIRCUT...

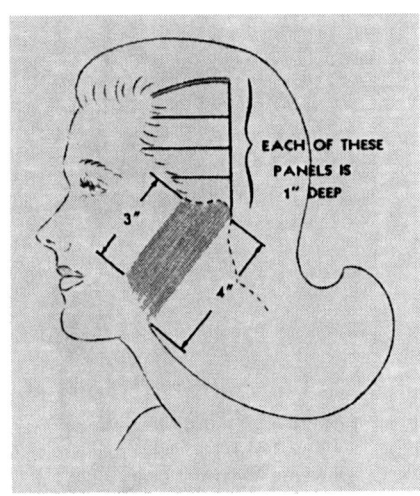

FIGURE 53. This diagram shows:

(a) The guide for cutting the left side hair. (The same as you used when giving the Baby Haircut.)

(b) How to part off the four panels of side hair prior to cutting. (The same as you did when giving the Baby Haircut.)

From a side view, notice how the length of the guide for cutting the side hair blends in one continuous line with the beautiful length and shape of the Middy Haircut in back.

FIGURE 54. Part off a panel of side hair one inch above the ear as shown below the heavy lines.

Cut and taper the hair in this panel to blend with the guide.

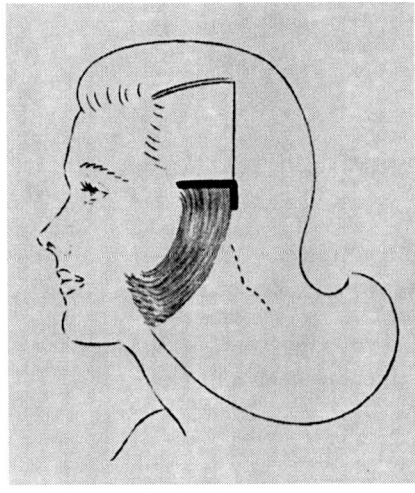

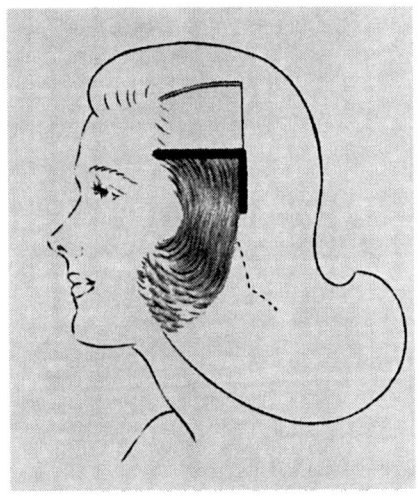

FIGURE 55. Part off another one inch deep panel of hair.

Cut and taper this hair to blend with the first panel of hair already cut.

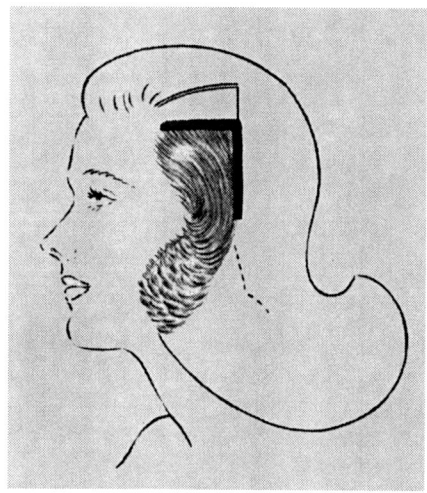

FIGURE 56. Part off another one inch deep panel of hair.

Cut and taper this hair to blend with the two panels already cut.

FIGURE 57. Bring down the remaining side hair and cut it to blend with the three panels already cut.

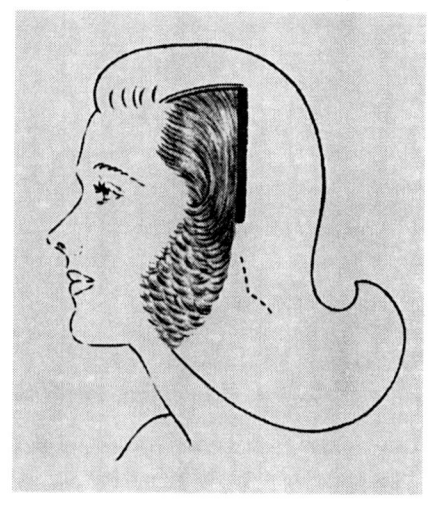

Next, cut and taper the right side hair exactly the same as you have done the left side.

Now that you have cut the nape, crown, and sides, all that remains to be cut is the top hair.

III. HOW TO CUT THE *Top Hair* WHEN GIVING A MIDDY HAIRCUT...

Turn to pages 26 and 27, and cut the top hair exactly as explained on those two pages.

THE *Middy Plus* HAIRCUT...

The Middy Plus Haircut differs from the Middy Haircut in only one respect; the nape and crown hair is shaped longer so it will blend with the Middy Plus guide.

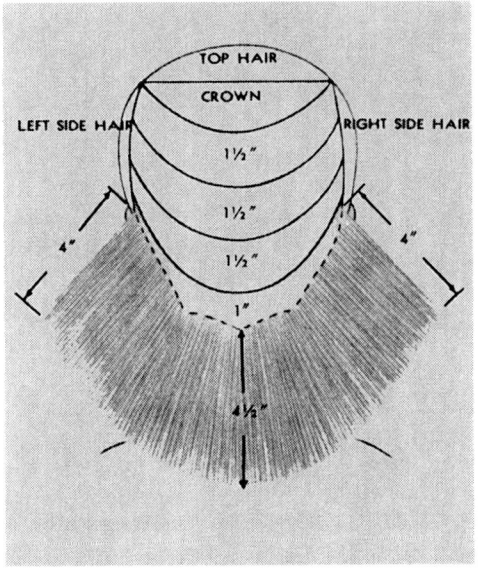

FIGURE 58. This diagram shows:

(a) The guide.
(b) How to part off the five panels of nape and crown hair to be cut. (The same as you did when you gave the Baby and Middy Haircuts.)

First, section off the top hair and pin it out of the way. (The same as you did when giving the Shingle, Shingle Plus, Baby, and Middy Haircuts.)

Next, make two crown-to-ear parts and pin the left and right side hair out of the way. (The same as you did when giving the Baby and Middy Haircuts.)

The guide is made by cutting the lowest center nape hair four and one-half inches in length. The lowest nape hair directly behind the upper part of the ears is four inches in length.

I. HOW TO CUT THE *Nape* AND *Crown Hair* WHEN GIVING A MIDDY PLUS HAIRCUT...

Follow the same cutting procedure you used when giving the Middy Haircut on pages 32 and 33, with this one exception: cut and taper the five panels of nape and crown hair to blend with the Middy Plus guide.

II. HOW TO CUT THE *Sides* WHEN GIVING A MIDDY PLUS HAIRCUT...

FIGURE 59. This diagram shows:

(a) The guide for cutting the left side hair. (The same as you used when giving the Baby and Middy Haircuts.)

(b) How to part off the four panels of side hair prior to cutting. (The same as you did when giving the Baby and Middy Haircuts.)

From a side view, notice how the length of the guide for cutting the side hair blends in one continuous line with the length and shape of the graceful lines of the Middy Plus Haircut in back.

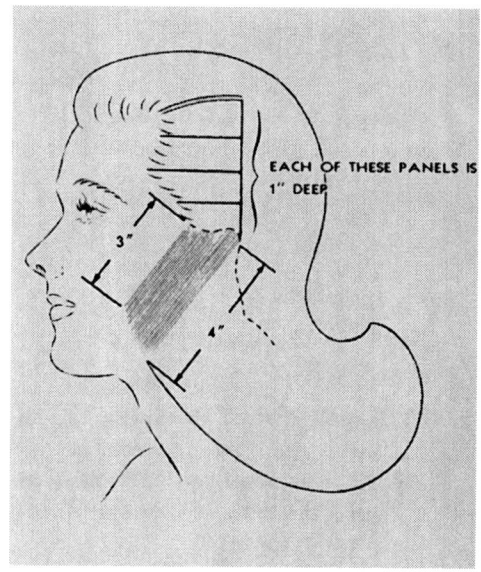

The instructions for cutting the left and right side hair when giving a Middy Plus Haircut are exactly the same as you used when cutting the sides for the Middy Haircut. So turn to pages 34 and 35, and cut the left and right side hair according to the instructions on those two pages.

III. HOW TO CUT THE *Top Hair* WHEN GIVING A MIDDY PLUS HAIRCUT...

Turn to pages 26 and 27, and cut the top hair according to the instructions on those pages.

THE *Long* HAIRCUT...

The Long Haircut differs from the Middy Plus Haircut only in one respect; the nape and crown hair is shaped longer so it will blend with the Long Haircut guide. If you are the Hollywood siren type, the Long Haircut with its graceful sloping lines will be the answer to your "I-want-to-be-glamorous" dreams.

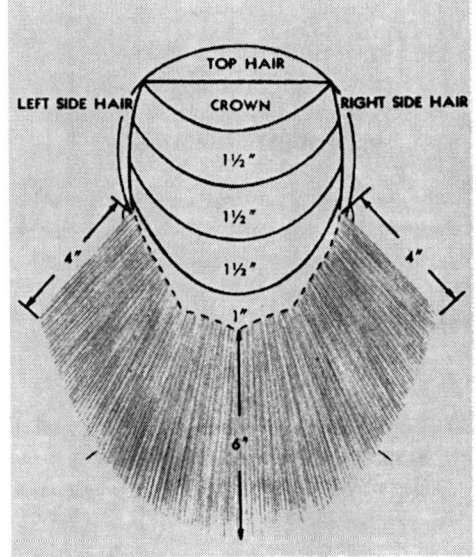

FIGURE 60. This diagram shows:

(a) The guide.

(b) How to part off the five panels of nape and crown hair to be cut. (The same as you did when you gave the Baby, Middy, and Middy Plus Haircuts.)

First, section off the top hair and pin it out of the way. (The same as you did when giving the Shingle, Shingle Plus, Baby, Middy, and Middy Plus Haircuts.)

Next, make two crown-to-ear parts and pin the left and right side hair out of the way. (The same as you did when giving the Baby, Middy, and Middy Plus Haircuts.)

The guide is made by cutting the lowest center nape hair six inches in length. The lowest nape hair directly behind the upper part of the ears is cut four inches in length.

I. HOW TO CUT THE *Nape* AND *Crown Hair* WHEN GIVING A LONG HAIRCUT...

Follow the same cutting procedure you used when giving the Middy Haircut on pages 32 and 33, with this one exception: Cut and taper the five panels of nape and crown hair to blend with the Long Haircut guide.

II. HOW TO CUT THE *Sides* WHEN GIVING A LONG HAIRCUT...

FIGURE 61. This diagram shows:

(a) The guide for cutting the left side hair. (The same as you used when giving the Baby, Middy, and Middy Plus Haircuts.)

(b) How to part off the four panels of side hair prior to cutting. (The same as you did when giving the Baby, Middy, and Middy Plus Haircuts.)

Observe how the length of the guide for cutting the side hair blends in one continuous line with the length and shape of the Long Haircut in back.

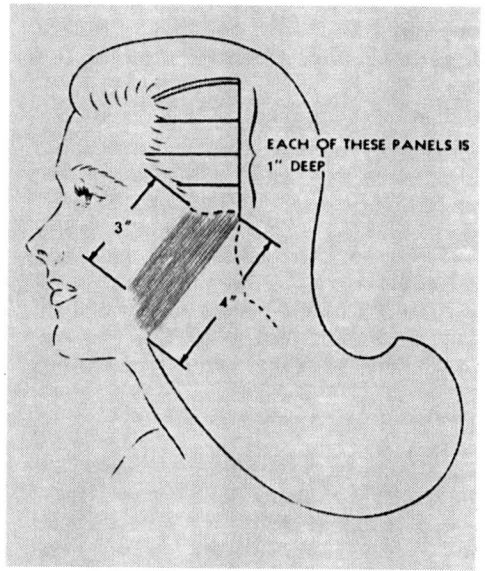

The instructions for cutting the left and right side hair when giving a Long Haircut are exactly the same as you followed when cutting the sides for the Middy Haircut. So turn to pages 34 and 35, and cut the left and right side hair according to the instructions on those two pages.

III. HOW TO CUT THE *Top Hair* WHEN GIVING A LONG HAIRCUT...

Turn to pages 26 and 27, and cut the top hair exactly as explained on those two pages.

Combination HAIRCUTS...

Suppose a hairstyle is desired that requires a top reverse roll. Obviously, all the Six Basic Haircuts would be too short on top to make a smooth reverse roll. The solution to this problem would be a Combination Haircut. The top hair would be cut to reverse roll length in a combination with any of the Six Basic Haircuts.

TOP REVERSE ROLL LENGTH

Divide the top hair into five one inch deep panels as you did when cutting the top hair for the Six Basic Haircuts.

Cut the top hair nearest the face six inches in length. As you work back gradually cut the hair shorter as illustrated in this sketch. The back portion of the top hair is cut five inches in length. The front top hair is longer because it has a greater distance to go to encircle the roll.

This sketch also shows a side view of all the guides for cutting the Six Basic Haircuts. Notice that the guide for the Shingle and Shingle Plus Haircuts is exactly the same at the sides and directly behind each ear.

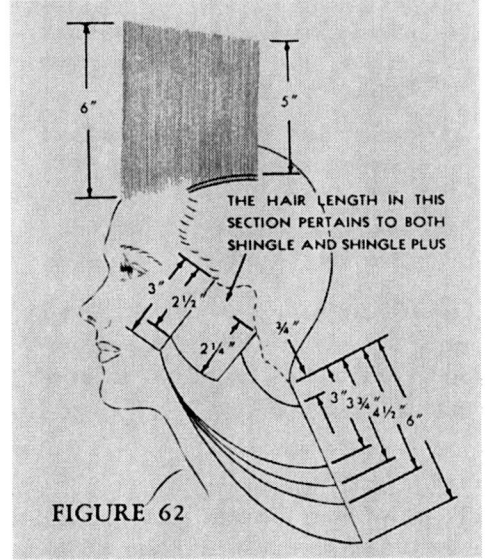

FIGURE 62

Also note that the guide for cutting the side hair is exactly the same for the Baby, Middy, Middy Plus and Long Haircuts, and that it blends in continuous lines with the four guides for cutting the nape and crown hair.

TOP HALF-WAVE REVERSE ROLL LENGTH

Cut the top hair nearest the face six and one-half inches in length. As you work back gradually cut the hair shorter. The back portion of the top hair is cut five and one-half inches in length.

TOP FULL WAVE REVERSE ROLL LENGTH

Cut the top hair nearest the face seven inches in length. As you work back gradually cut the hair shorter. The back portion of the top hair is cut six inches in length.

POMPADOUR LENGTH

Cut the top hair nearest the face eight inches in length. As you work back gradually cut the hair shorter. The back portion of the top hair is cut seven inches in length.

HALF-WAVE POMPADOUR LENGTH

Cut the top hair nearest the face eight and one-half inches in length. As you work back gradually cut the hair shorter. The back portion of the top hair is cut seven and one-half inches in length.

FULL WAVE POMPADOUR LENGTH

Cut the top hair nearest the face nine inches in length. As you work back gradually cut the hair shorter. The back portion of the top hair is cut eight inches in length.

SIDE REVERSE ROLL LENGTH

All the left and right side hair nearest the face is cut six inches in length. As you work back gradually cut the hair shorter as illustrated in this sketch. The back portion of the left and right side hair is cut five inches in length.

The side hair nearest the face is left longer because it has a greater distance to go to encircle the roll.

In this sketch, the lowest side hair is shown so you may compare the side reverse roll length with the length of the six guides.

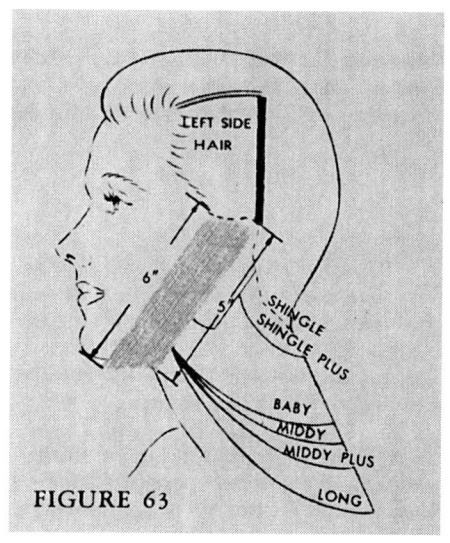

FIGURE 63

SIDE HALF-WAVE REVERSE ROLL LENGTH

All the left and right side hair nearest the face is cut six and one-half inches in length. As you work back gradually cut the hair shorter. The back portion of the left and right side hair is cut five and one-half inches in length.

SIDE FULL WAVE REVERSE ROLL LENGTH

All the left and right side hair nearest the face is cut seven inches in length. As you work back, gradually cut the hair shorter. The back portion of the left and right side hair is cut six inches in length.

TOP REVERSE ROLL LENGTH
TOP HALF-WAVE REVERSE ROLL LENGTH
TOP FULL WAVE REVERSE ROLL LENGTH
POMPADOUR LENGTH
HALF-WAVE POMPADOUR LENGTH
FULL WAVE POMPADOUR LENGTH

SIDE REVERSE ROLL LENGTH
SIDE HALF-WAVE REVERSE ROLL LENGTH
SIDE FULL WAVE REVERSE ROLL LENGTH

} These top and side haircut lengths may be used in combination with any of the Six Basic Haircuts.

HOW TO *Thin* HAIR...

When hair has been cut according to the Guide Method of Hairshaping, it is rarely necessary to thin the hair. However, some women do have hair that is too thick for proper styling, so it is necessary to know where to thin out the unwanted hair.

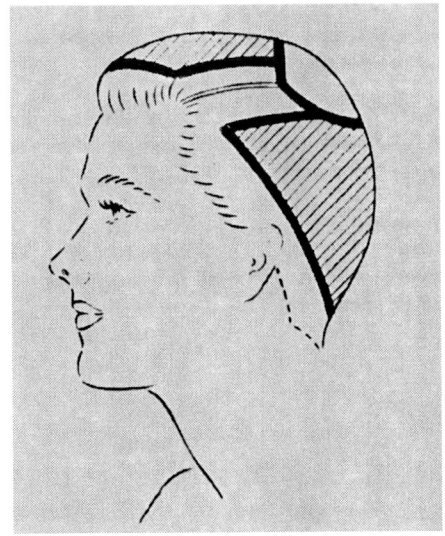

FIGURE 64. There are three popular tools that can be used to thin hair and they are: shears, thinning shears, and straight-edge razor. Whichever tool is used, the hair can be thinned to advantage only in the shaded areas.

In this sketch, the double line denotes a side part. If any other part is used, care should be taken not to thin hair closer than one inch to the part.

*G*ENERAL THINNING RULES...

1. Thin hair gradually. DO NOT thin hair out in large bunches because the hair will be difficult to catch when giving the permanent wave, and will be too unruly for proper styling.

2. Hair should not be thinned closer than one inch on either side of the part because the stubby ends would stand out unbecomingly.

3. Hair should not be thinned in the crown area for the same reason.

4. Hair should not be thinned directly over the ears or in the lower nape area because this hair is quite thin naturally.

5. Hair around the face should not be thinned within one inch of the hairline.

There are no set rules regarding the amount of hair to be thinned, but it is a good idea to follow the ancient cliche of all haircutters: "I can always take more off but I *can't* put it back on!!!"

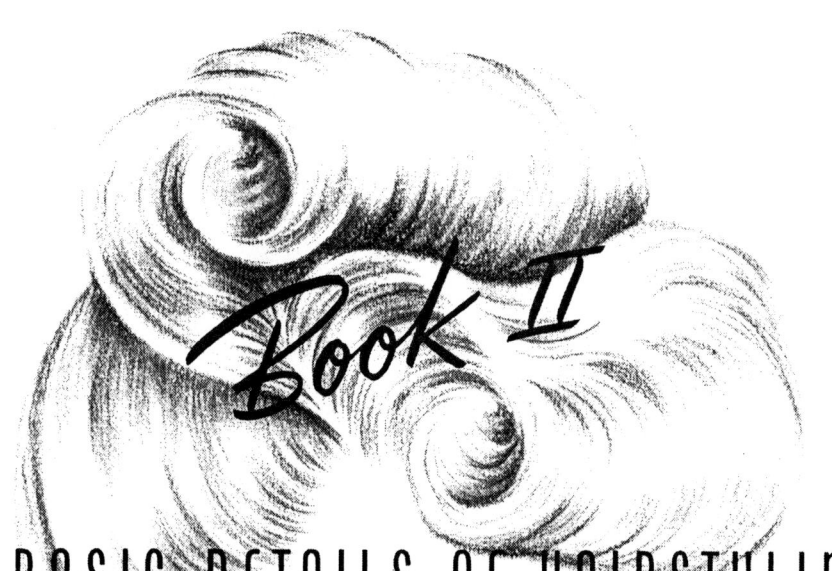

Book II

THE BASIC DETAILS OF HAIRSTYLING

Book II defines and illustrates the basic details which, when combined, produce our modern hairstyles.

BASIC *Hair Parts*

The importance of hair parts to successful hairstyling is usually underestimated. Many times the selection of a wrong part will ruin an otherwise beautiful hairdress. In this chapter, we will study the basic parts and their uses.

FIGURE 65. COWLICK PART:

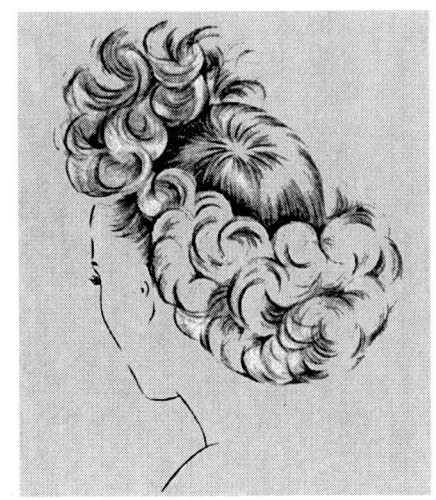

The starting point is the center of the cowlick. Imagine the cowlick as being a wheel, with the center of the cowlick as the hub, and the strands of hair as being the spokes. After locating the center of the cowlick, comb the hair away from it in the same directions as spokes diverge from a hub.

Notice in this Middy Haircut how the crown hair lies flat instead of buckling, and that the hairstyle is more becoming because the hair is properly distributed on the head.

A cowlick part may be used with any haircut, but is especially good when used with Baby or Middy Haircuts.

CENTER PART:

As we all know what a center part is, no sketch is necessary. It is important to know that a center part is very difficult to wear, and unless the model has an oval face or regular features, you will probably decide that some other kind of part would be more flattering.

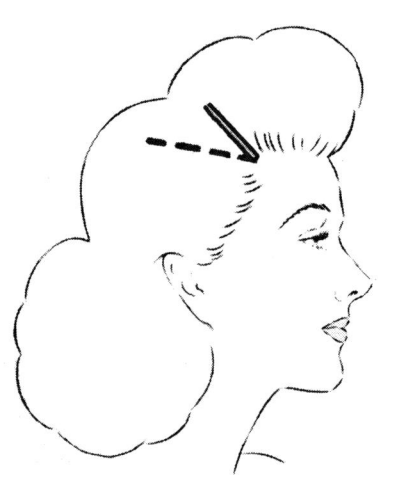

FIGURE 66. SIDE PART:

The side part, illustrated by the broken line, is the most popular of all parts because it may be used with many different styles, and is flattering to most women. If the side part is curved, it is called a ROUNDED SIDE PART. Side parts, or rounded side parts, may be used on either side of the head.

UP-DIAGONAL PART:

An up-diagonal part, illustrated by the double line, is recommended when the hair is thin because it allows some of the top and crown hair to fall on the small side.

If a diagonal part takes a downward direction, it is called a DOWN DIAGONAL PART.

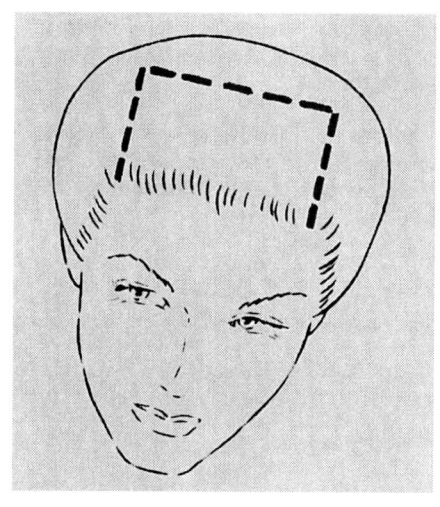

FIGURE 67. RECTANGULAR PART:

This basic part is usually used with rolls, pompadours, or bangs.

FIGURE 68. V PART:

A "V" part is somewhat of a novelty, and serves the same purpose as a rectangular part.

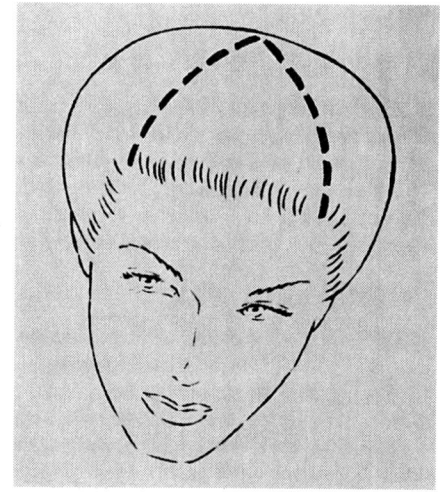

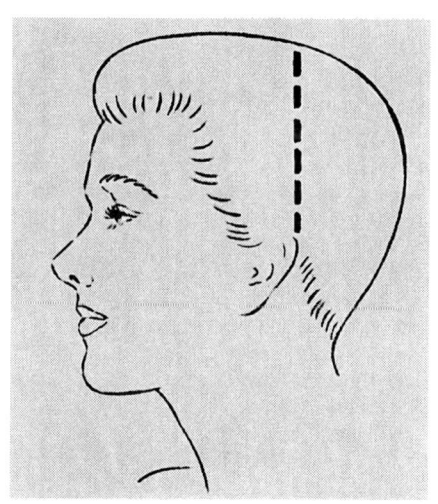

FIGURE 69. EAR-TO-EAR PART:

An ear-to-ear part extends from the upper back portion of one ear, over the top of the head, to the other ear.

This type of part is usually associated with all around-the-face reverse rolls or pompadours.

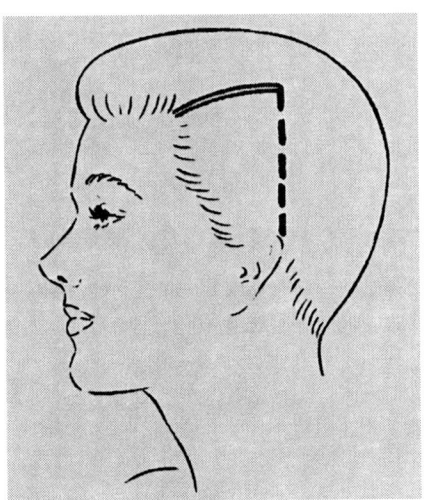

FIGURE 70.

CROWN-TO-EAR PART:

The dotted line illustrates a crown-to-ear part. It extends from the side of the crown to the ear.

In most cases a crown-to-ear part is used in combination with a side part. The side part in this sketch is indicated by the double line.

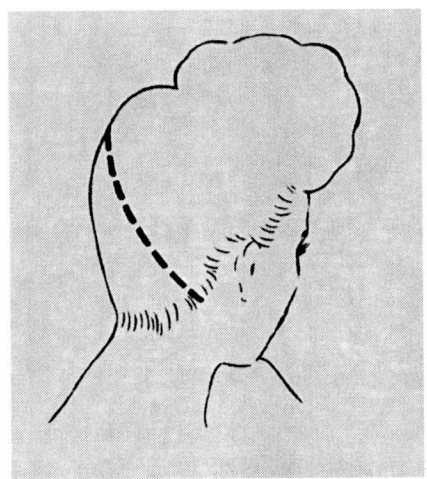

FIGURE 71.

BACK DIAGONAL PART:

Back diagonal parts were made popular by the French about 1938-39, but never gained much of a foothold in the United States as they are difficult to keep properly combed, and have a tendency to make the back of the head appear flat.

CENTER BACK PART:

This basic part extends from the center of the crown to the lowest center nape hair, and like the back diagonal part it quite often makes the back of the head appear flat. Because back diagonal parts and center back parts are difficult to comb, they are mostly used with formal hairstyles. The ten basic parts do not exhaust this subject, but they are the most common and will provide the student with a sound foundation so he or she may experiment with variations and combinations of parts.

GENERAL SUGGESTIONS REGARDING HAIR PARTS

To make side or center parts, comb the hair in the same direction as the part you have in mind. Next place the palm of your hand on the crown and press forward. The hair will automatically break into the most natural part.

If you are working with tinted or bleached hair and it has been some time since it was "touched up" avoid long parts that show where the hair has grown out. Many times it is possible to completely conceal parts by using bangs, rolls, flowers or hair ornaments.
If there are scars or bumps on the head, select parts that do not expose them.
Parts are interesting and essential to creative hairstyling, so spend considerable time experimenting with different parts and combinations of parts.

Further information on the correct use of parts for the different face types and for facial irregularities is given in Book III.

BASIC *Waves*

Most hairstyles are created by using waves and curls. In this chapter the three basic waves will be illustrated, and in the following chapter curls will be discussed.

One wave is composed of two ridges going in opposite directions. When setting a wave, do not force the hair. *Do* follow the natural or permanent wave tendencies of the hair, and the finished result will not appear artificial, will last longer, and will be easier to comb. Try setting the waves with a slight curve and you will find that they will be more beautiful than absolutely straight waves.

FIGURE 72.
THE THREE BASIC WAVES

1. SHADOW WAVE

Shadow waves are wide and the ridges are not sharp. Because this type of wave is subtle and natural looking, it is beautiful and flattering.

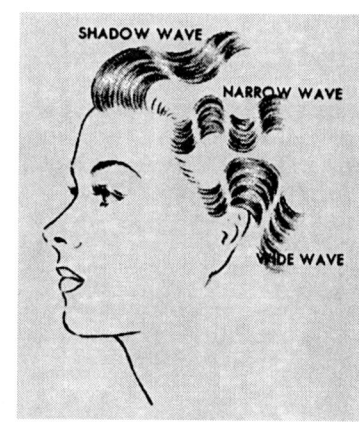

2. NARROW WAVE

The ridges of a narrow wave are sharp and close together. Some types of fine hair do not hold a shadow or wide wave, so a narrow wave must be used even though it is not as beautiful.

3. WIDE WAVE

Wide waves are becoming to most people and should be used extensively. The ridges are just a little sharper than found in a shadow wave.

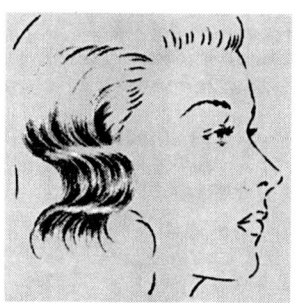

The three basic waves may take either a horizontal, vertical, or diagonal direction.

FIGURE 73. HORIZONTAL

Any basic wave that takes a direction parallel to the horizon is said to be horizontal.

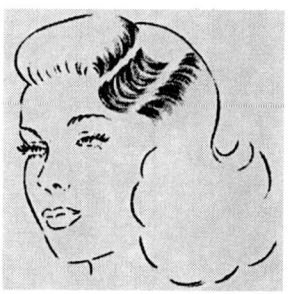

FIGURE 74. VERTICAL

Any basic wave that takes a straight up-and-down direction is said to be vertical.

FIGURE 75. DIAGONAL

Any basic wave that takes a direction between horizontal and vertical is said to be diagonal.

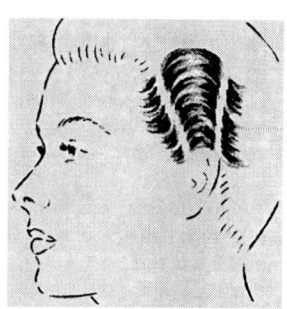

BASIC *Half-Waves*

A half-wave is just what it appears to be—it is one half of a full wave, and has one ridge. A half-wave may take either a horizontal, vertical or diagonal direction.

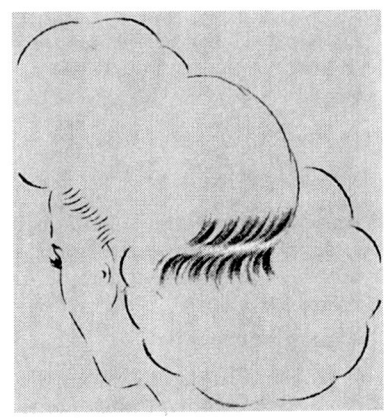

FIGURE 76.

HORIZONTAL HALF-WAVE

Here we see the most popular placement of a horizontal half-wave. It molds the nape hair to the back of the head and provides a "foundation" for the curls on the neck.

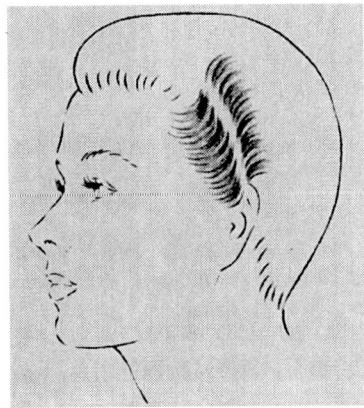

FIGURE 77.

VERTICAL UP HALF-WAVE

The up half-wave takes a straight up-and-down direction so it is said to be a vertical up half-wave.

When a vertical up half-wave is followed by curls, it is one of the most flattering and popular details found in modern hairstyling.

If the half-wave in this sketch took a down direction, it would be called a VERTICAL DOWN HALF-WAVE.

FIGURE 78.

DIAGONAL HALF-WAVE

A half-wave that takes a direction between a horizontal and vertical is called a diagonal half-wave.

This drawing shows how a diagonal half-wave looks when placed on the back of the head.

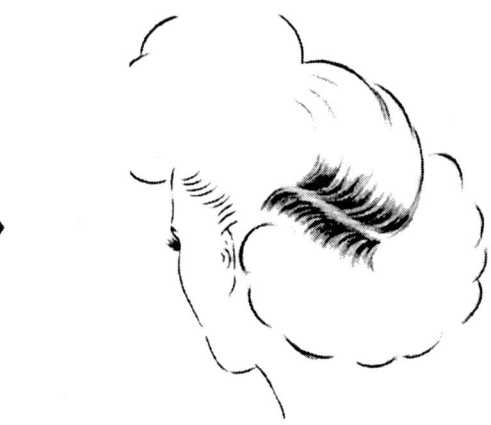

FIGURE 79.

When a diagonal half-wave is placed over the ears, it looks like this illustration. The author considers the diagonal half-wave over the ears one of the most flattering and becoming details that has ever been designed for the younger set.

Study this illustration carefully. It looks simple, but it is one of the most difficult hair details to execute.

Step-by-step instructions for setting a diagonal half-wave are given on page 104.

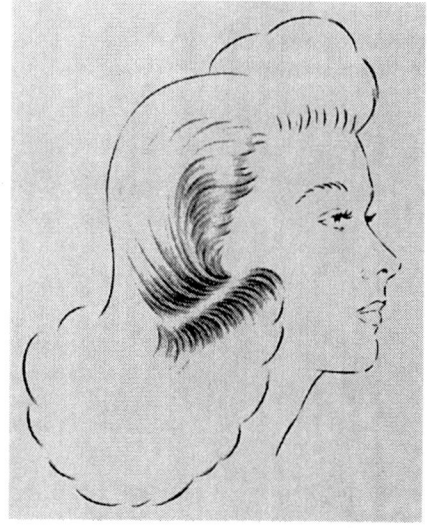

FIGURE 80.

STAND-UP HALF-WAVE

The trick of setting the stand-up half-wave is this: the top hair near the hairline is combed against the natural wave tendency so that it almost stands on end. Then the half-wave is pushed into place and held into position by three or four bobby pins while it dries. The bobby pins are inserted one-fourth inch below the ridge.

The stand-up half-wave is becoming to most women, and may be followed by curls, reverse roll, or pompadour.

The stand-up half-wave may take either a left or right direction. In this illustration it takes a left direction.

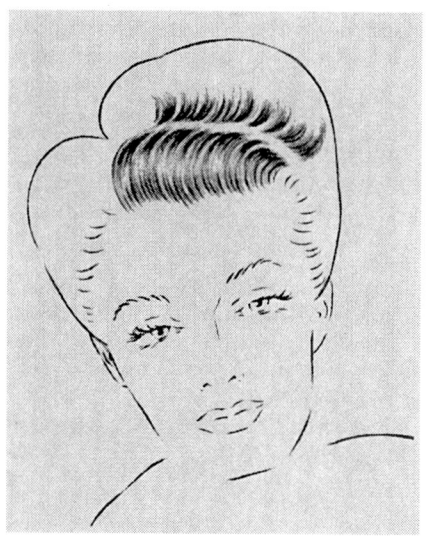

BASIC *Curls*

There are two basic curls—the pin curl and the sculpture curl. Both pin curls and sculpture curls are composed of two sections:

> **BASE:** The beginning of the curl. The base indicates the direction the curl takes.
>
> **LOOPS:** The number of loops to make a curl depends on the size of the curl, the thickness of the hair, and the length of the hair.

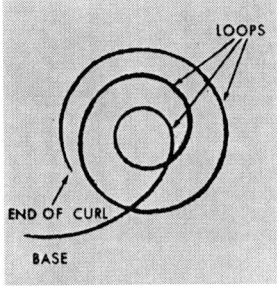

FIGURE 81. PIN CURL

This basic curl is by far the most commonly used and is the easiest to do. It is made by winding strands of hair around the finger. Each loop is *outside* of the last loop and the ends of the hair are on the *outside* of the curl.

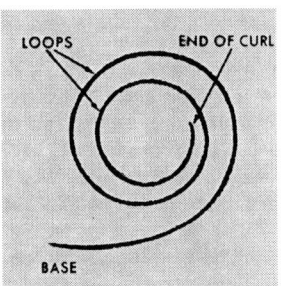

FIGURE 82. SCULPTURE CURL

The sculpture curl is the finest curl known and is used by all master hairstylists. It follows the natural tendency of the hair, stays in longer, and the finished effect is more beautiful and professional looking than any other type of curl.

The chief characteristics of the sculpture curl are: each loop is *inside* of the last loop, and the ends of the hair are on the *inside* of the curl. Step-by-step instructions showing how the sculpture curl is made will be given later in this chapter.

The author prefers and encourages the use of the sculpture curl, but if you choose to use the pin curl, or any other type of curl, you are assured that the setting instructions in this volume will apply equally well to all kinds of curls.

FIGURE 83. SYMBOL FOR A CURL

For the sake of clarity and simplicity of instruction, the symbol shown here will be used throughout to denote a curl. The base immediately indicates the direction the curl takes. Whenever you see the symbols for curls you will notice that they are numbered. It is important that you make the curls in the order numbered as this prevents the completed curls from getting in the way while you work.

On the following pages curl symbols will be used in the setting instructions to show where the curls are placed, and the direction the curls take to achieve a certain result.

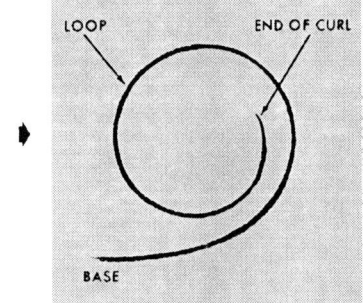

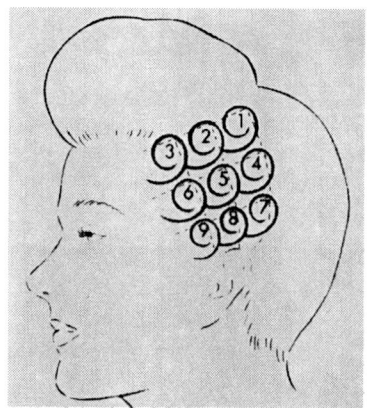

FIGURE 84. HOW CURLS ARE MADE FROM BLOCKS OF HAIR

THE FIRST STEP

Part off a block of hair *about* an inch square. (Blocks may be made either larger or smaller if desired.) The dotted lines denote the blocks.

THE SECOND STEP

Now mold the hair in the block into a curl, and secure it with hairpins or bobby pin until dry.

It will be noted that the curls *are not* placed in the center of the blocks. The hair purposely overlaps the blocks in order that all the hair will be curling in the same direction, thus preventing any buckling in the finished detail.

FIGURE 85. HOW CURLS ARE MADE WHEN THEY FOLLOW THE RIDGE OF A WAVE

Whenever you see symbols for curls you will assume that the curls are made from nearly square blocks except when the curls follow the ridge of a wave.

If the curls follow the ridge of a wave, the blocks will be one-fourth of an inch from the ridge as shown by the dotted line. Study this illustration carefully so you will know how the curls are placed in relation to the blocks.

Curls "1" to "4" inclusive are made from blocks one-fourth of an inch from the ridge and one inch deep.

Curls "5" through "8" are made from blocks that are almost square.

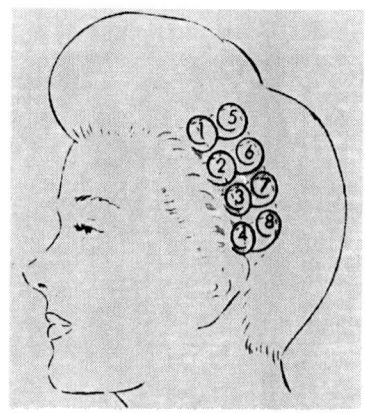

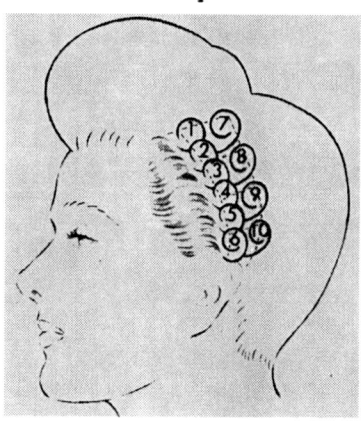

FIGURE 86. OVERLAPPING CURLS

In many cases where curls follow the ridge of a wave, the curls will overlap because the hair is long or thick. This drawing shows how the overlapping curls ("1" through "6") are made from blocks one-fourth of an inch from the ridge. Notice that these blocks are a little less than one inch deep.

When making overlapping curls it is imperative that you make the curls in the order numbered so the completed curls will not be in the way while you work.

HOW TO MAKE *Sculpture Curls*

Especially now that permanent waves can be given by the use of curls, it is even more important that we know how to make perfect sculpture curls. After hairstyling contests and demonstrations, students and beauticians have expressed their desire to learn the author's method of making sculpture curls. In response to those requests, photographs of each step in making sculpture curls are given.

FIGURE 87. Part off a block of hair about one inch square. The blocks will vary in size depending on the degree of tightness or looseness desired.

Then comb the hair in the same direction that the detail will take when the curls are dried and combed out.

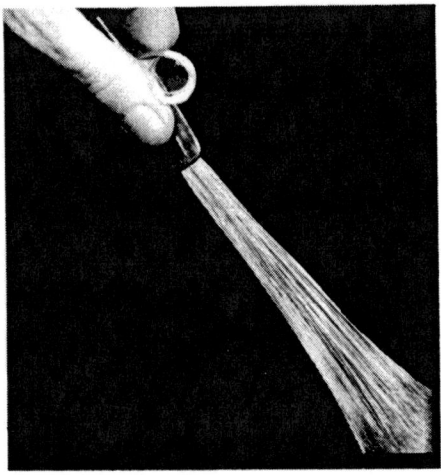

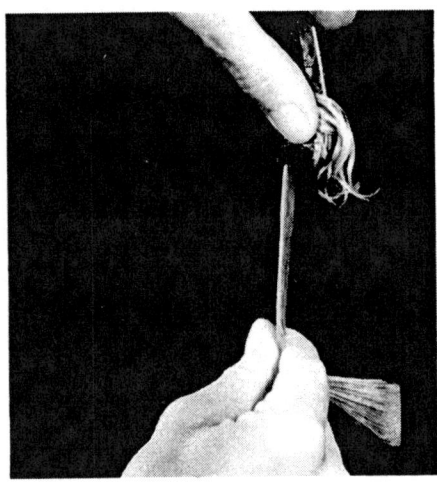

FIGURE 88. Comb the strands of hair with a twisting motion of the comb in order to find the permanent, or natural wave tendency.

FIGURE 89. This shows how the hair will look when the permanent, or natural wave tendency has been found.

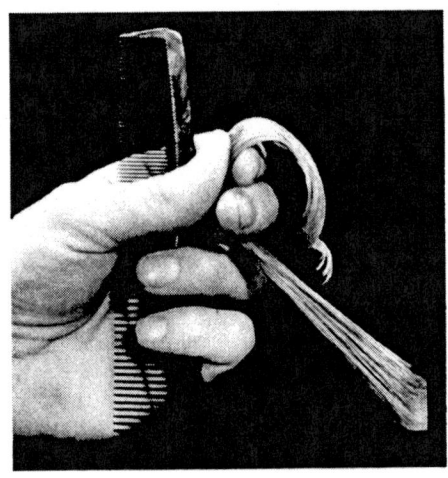

FIGURE 90. Following the permanent or natural wave tendency, form the outside loop.

Then fold the second loop *inside* of the outside loop.

Continue to fold all succeeding loops inside of the last loop made.

The ends of the strands are placed in the center of the sculpture curl.

It will be noted that the sculpture curl is started at the base rather than starting at the end and working toward the base. Attention is also called to the fact that the strands of hair are not wound around the finger in pin curl fashion.

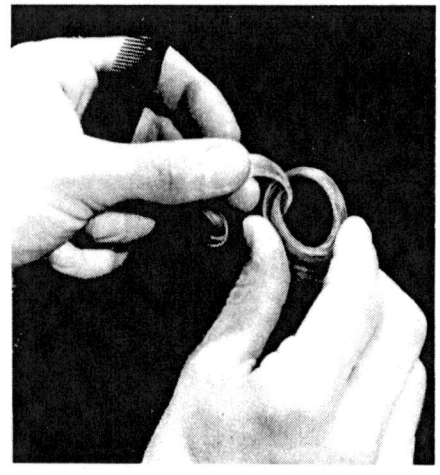

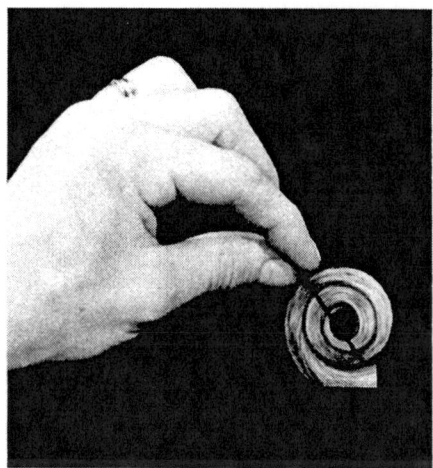

FIGURE 91. Bobby or hairpins are inserted to hold the sculpture curl in place until dry. Bobby pins are recommended because they are faster (use only one) and do not allow the curl to slip out of position during the drying time.

To avoid ridges on the curl *do not* slide the bobby pin over the curl. *Do* hold the bobby pin open until it completely covers the curl.

BASIC *Rolls*

Rolls are made from curls, or from a combination of curls and waves or half-waves. Refer to the haircutting chapter for the best hair lengths for each of the basic rolls.

These are the six basic rolls used on the top and sides of the head.

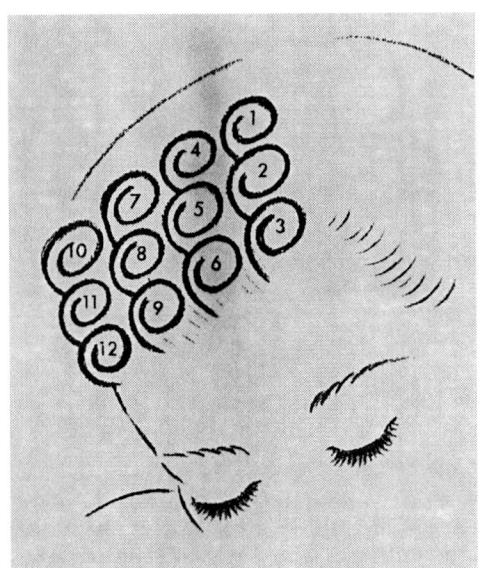

FIGURE 92.

1. TOP REVERSE ROLL
(setting instructions)

Make a rectangular part. The larger the rectangular part, the larger the roll will be.

Next, subdivide the rectangular part into blocks about an inch square, and you are ready to mold the curls.

Comb the hair in each block straight back and mold the curls in the order numbered.

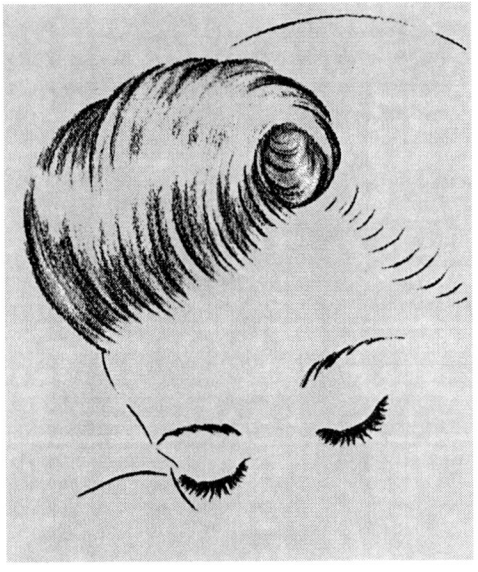

FIGURE 93.

TOP REVERSE ROLL
(combed out)

After drying, all the curls in the section are combed out together in a back direction over the palm of the hand, and the ends are turned under.

This type of roll is quite severe and is not becoming to very many women.

FIGURE 94.

2. TOP HALF-WAVE REVERSE ROLL
(setting instructions)

Make the half-wave, and mold the curls starting with curl numbered 1.

As in all cases where curls follow the ridge of a half-wave, the first row of curls is made from blocks one-fourth of an inch back of the ridge as explained in the Curl Chapter.

When the hair is thick or long, the first row of curls following the ridge will overlap as they do in this illustration.

Two rows of curls are usually sufficient to make a top half-wave reverse roll, but three rows of curls may be used if an extra large roll is desired.

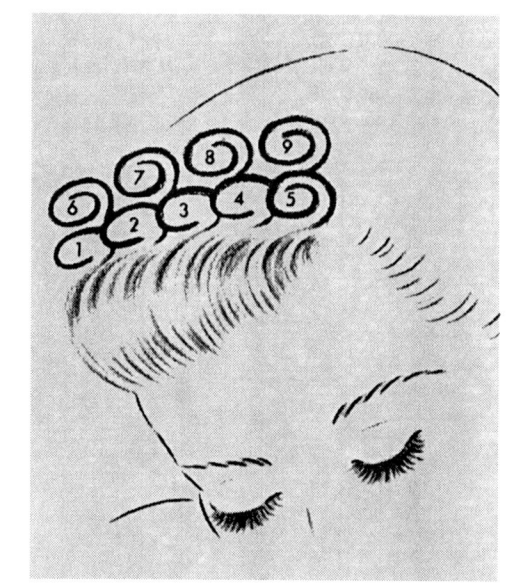

FIGURE 95.

TOP HALF-WAVE REVERSE ROLL
(combed out)

After drying, the half-wave and all the curls in the rectangular part are combed out together in a back direction over the palm of the hand, and the ends are turned under.

Because the top half-wave reverse roll is flattering and easy to execute, it is suggested that you use it quite often in your styling.

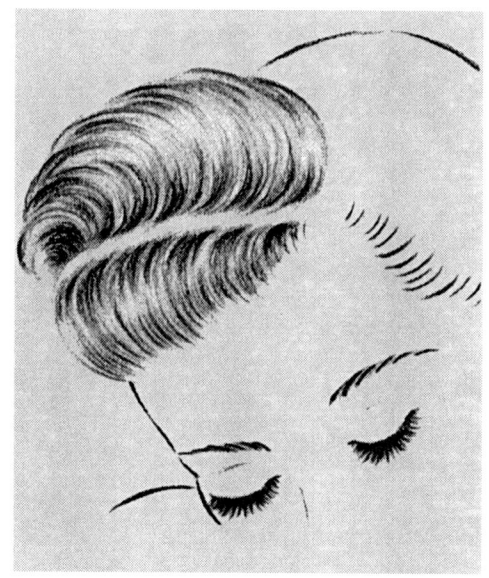

3. TOP FULL WAVE REVERSE ROLL

This type reverse roll is beautiful if properly executed. The important thing to remember is to make the wave curve and vary in width as shown in the sketches below.

There are two ways to do a top full wave reverse roll. The first and easiest method is to make one complete wave followed by two rows of curls. The second method produces a softer looking roll and is more difficult, so the advanced setting instructions will be given.

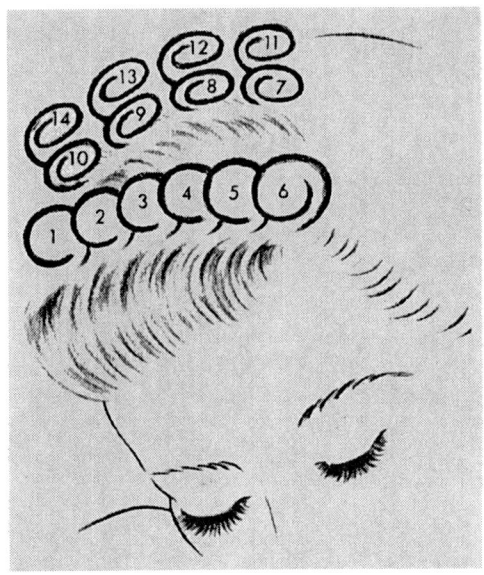

FIGURE 96.

TOP FULL WAVE REVERSE ROLL
(advanced setting instructions)

First a half-wave is made followed by one row of overlapping curls.

Then the second ridge of the wave is made followed by one or two rows of curls. Two rows of curls make a larger roll.

Be sure to make the curls in the order numbered.

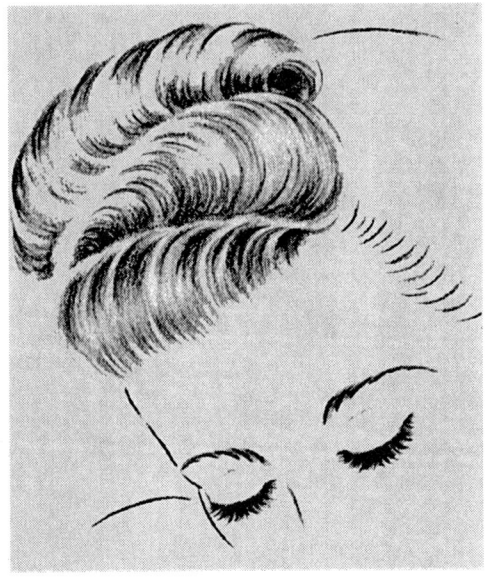

FIGURE 97.

TOP FULL WAVE REVERSE ROLL
(combed out)

After drying, the wave and curls are thoroughly brushed and combed out together. The ends are then turned under.

In the event the advanced setting instructions were followed, you will discover that much brushing and combing will cause the first row of curls to blend in with the second ridge, making it appear deep and natural looking.

FIGURE 98.

4. SIDE REVERSE ROLL

(setting instructions)

First, section off the side hair.

Then, working with blocks about an inch square, comb the strands of hair in a back and up direction and mold the curls in the order numbered.

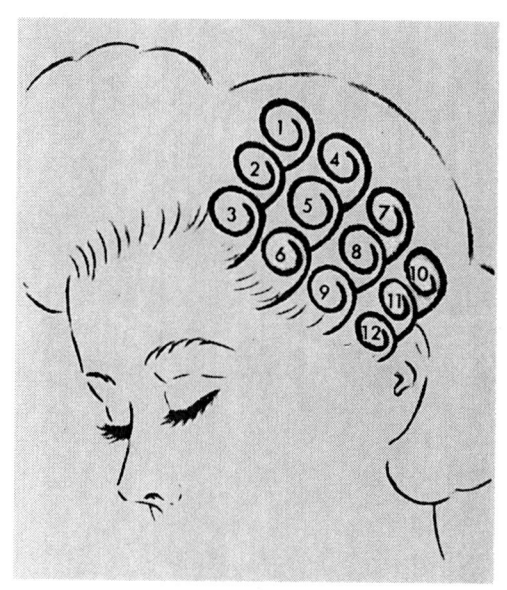

FIGURE 99.

SIDE REVERSE ROLL (combed out)

After drying, all the curls are combed out together in a back and up direction. The ends of the hair are then rolled under.

Rats may be used to advantage if the hair is thin and a larger roll is desired.

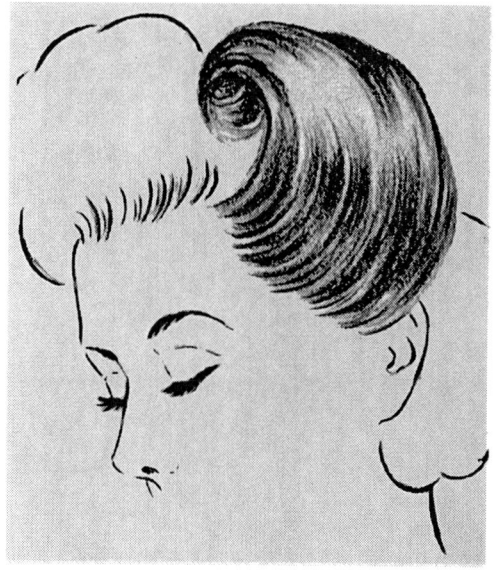

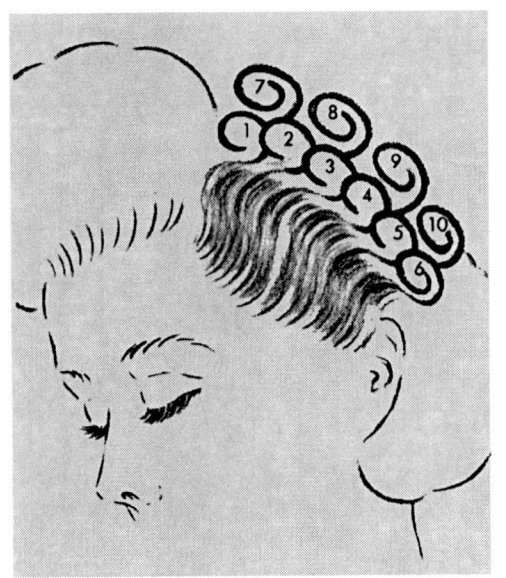

FIGURE 100.

5. SIDE HALF-WAVE REVERSE ROLL
(setting instructions)

Make a down half-wave followed by two rows of up curls as illustrated. Be sure to make the curls in the order numbered.

Notice that the first row of curls overlap in this drawing, but in some cases where the hair is short but not thick, the curls will not overlap.

There are two tricks in making beautiful side half-wave reverse rolls, and they are: first, comb the side hair in an upward direction before making the down half-wave. This will give the hairstyle a "lift" when it is combed out. Secondly, set the down half-wave so that it has a curve instead of being straight. Rounded half-waves are always more becoming than straight half-waves.

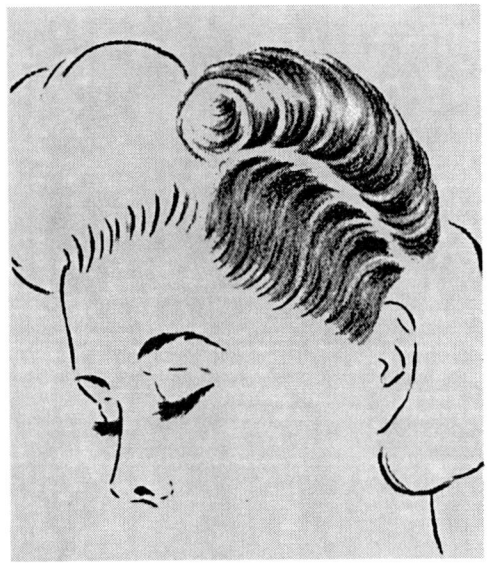

FIGURE 101.

SIDE HALF-WAVE REVERSE ROLL
(combed out)

After drying, the half-wave and all the curls are combed out together in a back and up direction. The ends are turned under.

6. SIDE FULL WAVE REVERSE ROLL

This type of reverse roll can be made by two different methods. The first and easiest way is to make one complete wave followed by two rows of up curls. The second and more advanced method is more difficult to do, so the advanced setting instructions will be given.

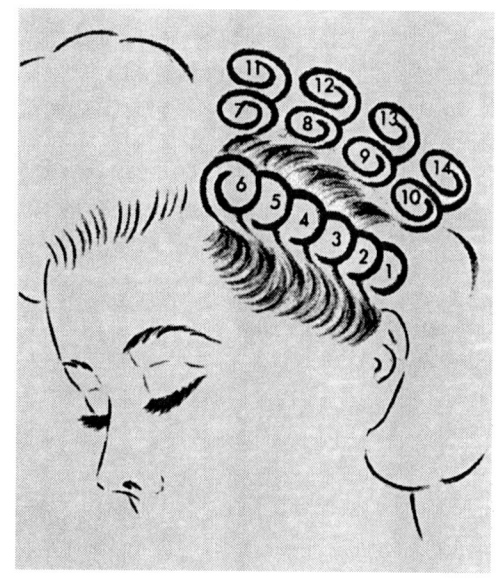

FIGURE 102.

SIDE FULL WAVE REVERSE ROLL
(advanced setting instructions)

Make an up half-wave, followed by one row of down overlapping curls. Then the second ridge of the wave is made followed by two rows of up curls.

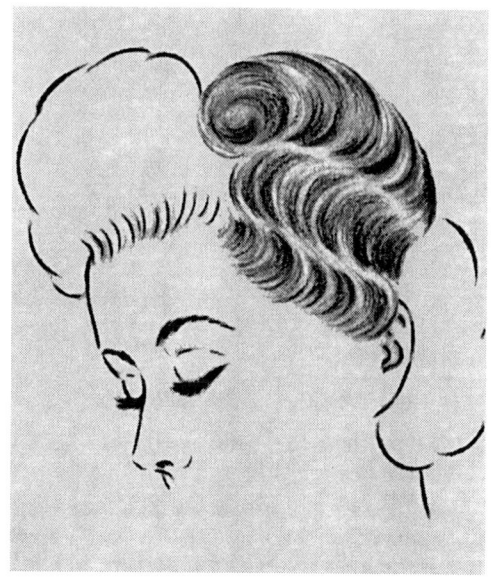

FIGURE 103.

SIDE FULL WAVE REVERSE ROLL
(combed out)

After drying, the wave and curls are thoroughly brushed and combed out together. The ends are then turned under.

If the advanced setting instructions were followed, you will discover that much brushing and combing will cause the first row of curls to blend in with the second ridge, making it appear deep and natural looking.

The six basic rolls which you have learned in this chapter were combed back and the ends under, and for this reason are called reverse rolls.

Without changing the setting, the six basic rolls can be combed forward and under. They would then be called:

> TOP FORWARD ROLL
> TOP HALF-WAVE FORWARD ROLL
> TOP FULL WAVE FORWARD ROLL
>
> SIDE FORWARD ROLL
> SIDE HALF-WAVE FORWARD ROLL
> SIDE FULL WAVE FORWARD ROLL

So there can be no doubt in your mind as to what forward rolls are, one of the six forward rolls will be illustrated.

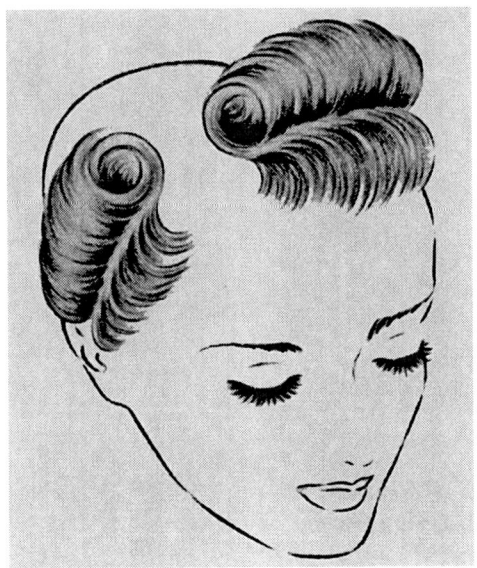

FIGURE 104.

TOP HALF-WAVE FORWARD ROLL

Set the top hair the same as you did for a top half-wave reverse roll. After the hair is dry comb the roll forward and under to achieve this effect.

(Note: The direction the top half-wave takes is determined by the personal preference of the patron and the way the top hair grows near the hairline. In this illustration, the top half-wave goes to the right, and in Figure 95, the top half-wave goes to the left.)

ROLL VARIATIONS

After you have learned the six basic rolls, you will be able to design and execute a great number of roll variations. It is impractical in this chapter to show all the roll variations, but one example will be given.

SIDE UP HALF-WAVE FORWARD ROLL

In Figure 104, the side hair was set with an up half-wave followed by two rows of down curls. After drying, the side hair is combed forward and under to achieve this roll variation. In Book IV several roll variations are illustrated.

BASIC *Pompadours*

There are three basic pompadours, and the setting instructions are exactly the same as for top reverse roll, top half-wave reverse roll, and top full wave reverse roll. The only difference between the reverse rolls made from top hair, and pompadours is this: The top hair used for pompadours is longer, as explained in the haircut chapter, and pompadours stand up higher.

FIGURE 105.

1. STRAIGHT BACK POMP

Since the setting instructions are exactly the same as for the top reverse roll, page 54, they will not be repeated here.

The straight back pomp is very severe and is not flattering to many women.

In this and the other two basic pompadours, tease the hair or insert rats to give additional height and fullness.

To achieve this effect, the sides are set in curls for side reverse rolls. See page 57 for setting instructions.

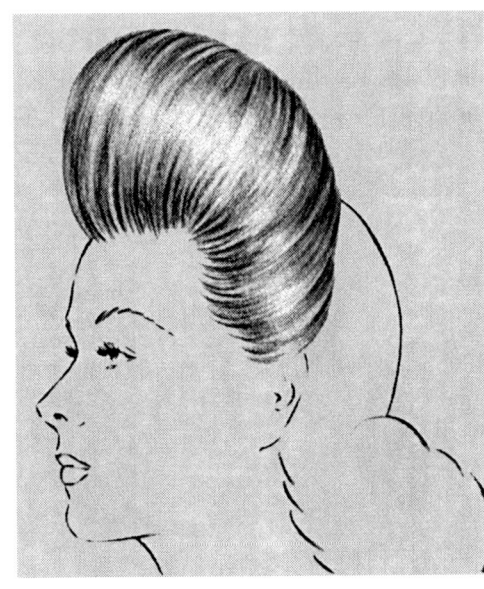

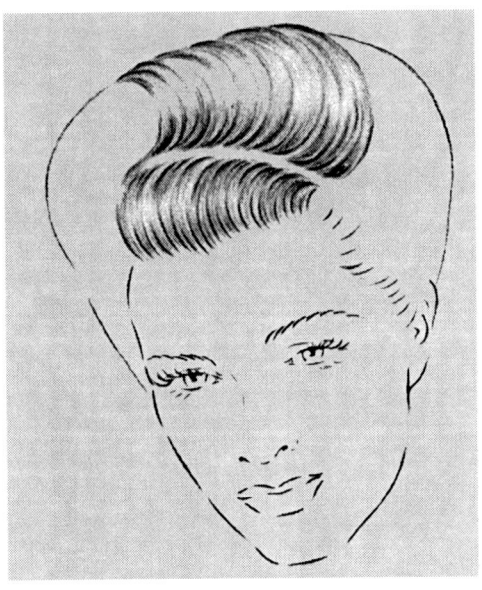

FIGURE 106.

2. HALF-WAVE POMP

The setting instructions are exactly the same as for the top half-wave reverse roll, page 55.

The half-wave pomp is much softer looking than the straight-back pomp and has at times been quite popular.

FIGURE 107.

3. FULL WAVE POMP

The setting instructions are exactly the same as for the top full wave reverse roll, page 56.

Many older women prefer the full wave pomp, and since it seems to suggest the elderly matron group, it is not a favorite with young women.

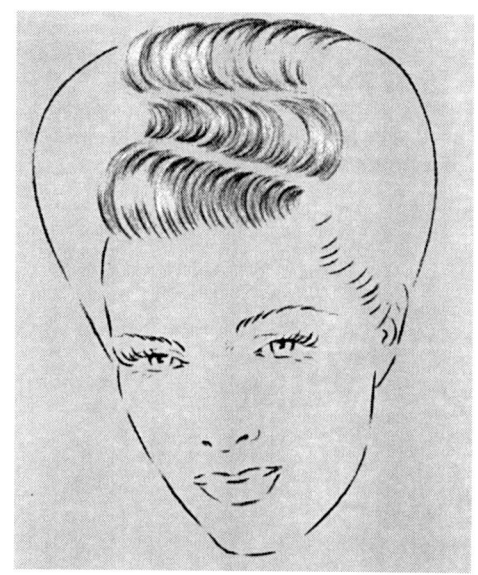

FIGURE 108.

FINISHED HAIRSTYLE SHOWING FULL WAVE POMP

This hairdress is presented to show how the full wave pomp blends with the side hair.

To set the right and left side hair, make a vertical up half-wave followed by two rows of large, down curls.

After drying, comb the top hair, right side hair, and left side hair together and turn the ends under.

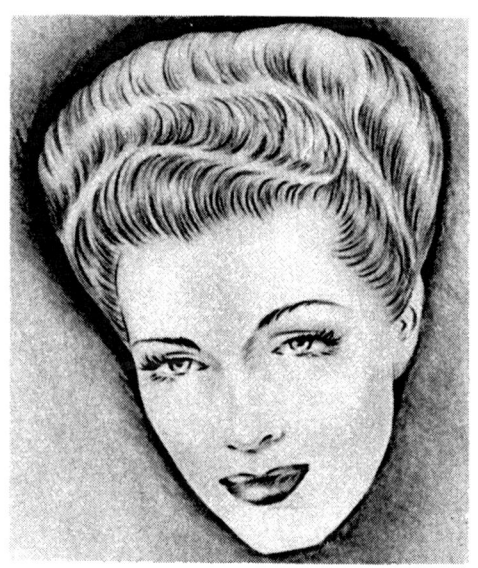

BASIC *Bangs*

The most important requisite of beautiful bangs is rhythm, so by all means, avoid straight or square lines. Strive for softness.

There are six basic bangs, and they may be used in combination with almost all the other hairstyle details.

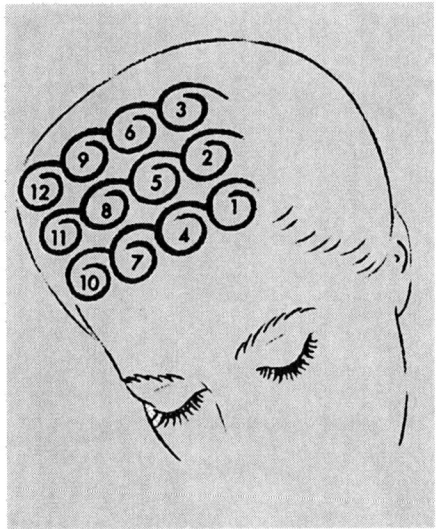

FIGURE 109.

1. FLUFF BANGS
(setting instructions)

Make a rectangular part.

The top hair used for the bangs is cut from three to four inches in length, and is set in forward curls as illustrated.

Do not attempt fluff bangs if the top hair is over four inches long because it will fall into curls instead of fluffing.

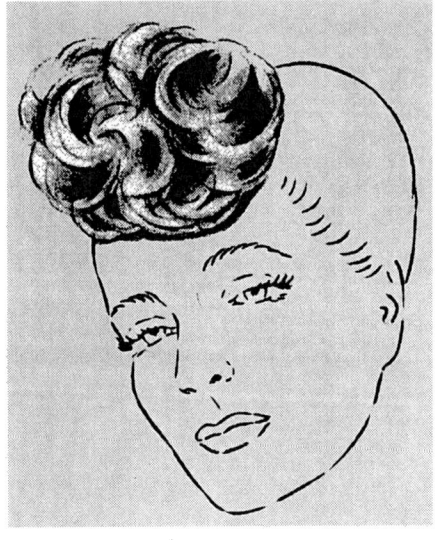

FIGURE 110.

FLUFF BANGS (combed out)

Simply run the comb through the curls, and allow the hair to fall into a casual fluff.

2. FORWARD ROLL BANGS (setting instructions)

The top hair used in this type of bangs should be five inches long in front, and seven inches long in back.

Make a rectangular part, and set the hair in forward curls the same as you did when setting the hair for fluff bangs. (See Figure 109 for the setting instructions).

FIGURE 111.

FORWARD ROLL BANGS (combed out)

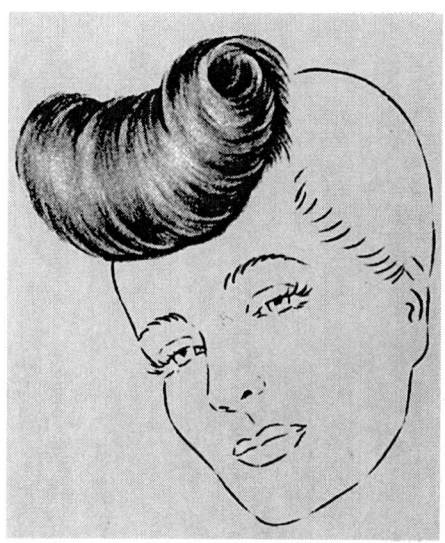

Comb and brush all the curls out together. Then comb the hair forward and over the palm of one hand. Turn the ends under.

Particular care should be taken to avoid a straight across line as this would make the top of the head appear flat and uninteresting. As in all bangs, a curved line is more becoming than a straight across line.

To achieve the high and irregular outline as in this sketch, comb the hair over a rat or tease the hair.

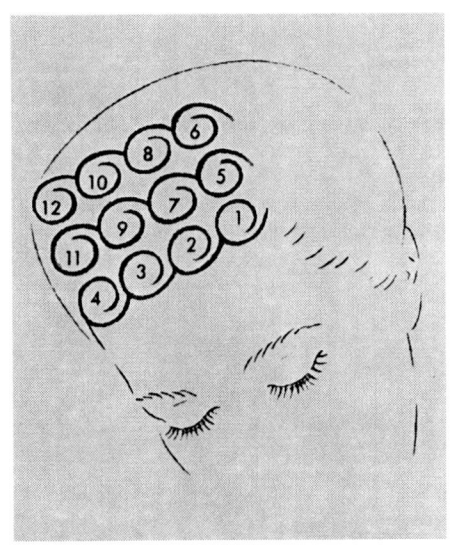

FIGURE 112.

3. HALF-WAVE BANGS
(setting instructions)

Make a rectangular part.

The top hair used in the bangs is four inches long in front and six inches long in back. (This is the top hair length of all Basic Haircuts *except* the Baby Haircut)

Set the curls as illustrated in this sketch.

Special attention is called to the fact that the curls in the first row are turned backward, while the other two rows of curls are turned forward.

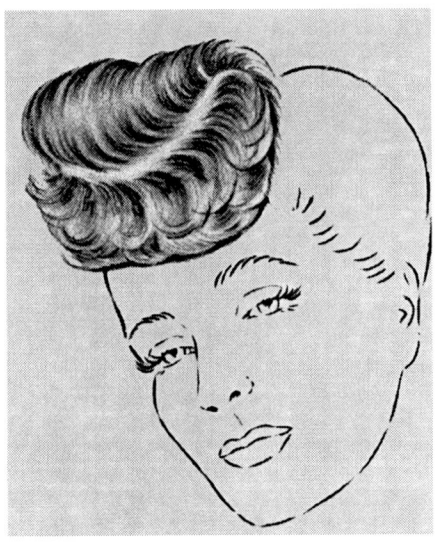

FIGURE 113.

HALF-WAVE BANGS (combed out)

All the curls are vigorously combed and brushed out together. Then comb the hair over the palm of one hand and push the half-wave into the hair. Since the ends of the hair are short, they will fall casually.

If the bangs are flat because the hair does not have enough body, use a rat, or tease the hair.

As in all bangs, be sure to arrange the hair in subtle, soft curves.

FIGURE 114.

4. FULL WAVE BANGS
(setting instructions)

Make a rectangular part.

The top hair should be five and one-half inches long in front, and seven and one-half inches long in back.

Set the curls as illustrated in this sketch.

The front two rows of curls are turned backward, and curls in the third row are turned forward.

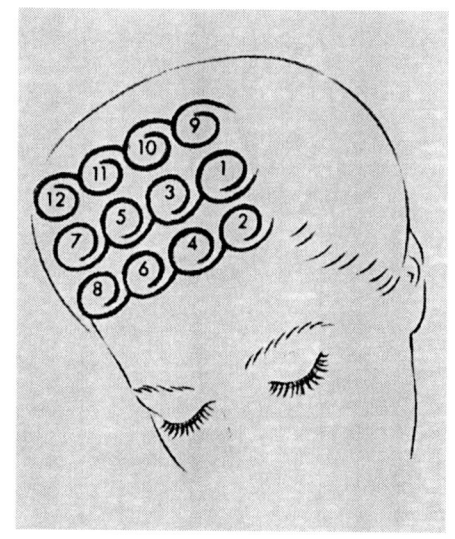

FIGURE 115.

FULL WAVE BANGS (combed out)

It is essential with this type of bangs that the curls be thoroughly brushed and combed. The more you brush, the deeper and more natural the wave becomes.

Comb the hair over the palm of one hand and push the wave into the bang so it takes a graceful curve. Turn the ends under.

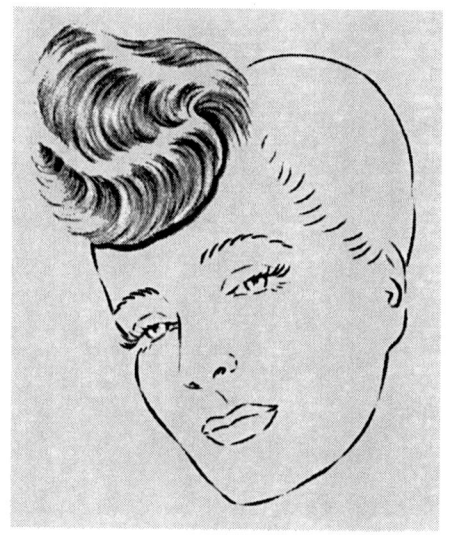

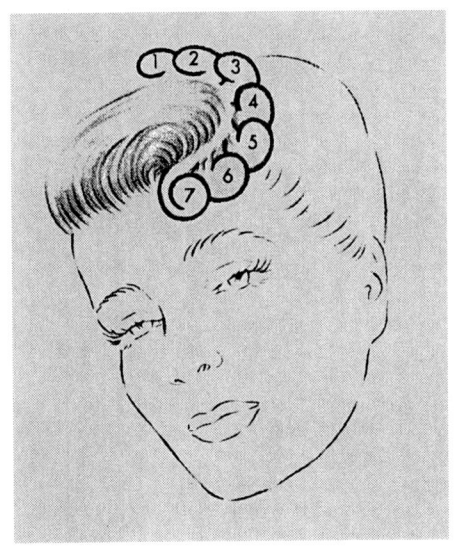

FIGURE 116.

5. FRENCH BANGS
(setting instructions)

The secret of successful French Bangs is to comb the top hair almost straight back off the forehead, and then swirl the hair forward to make the half-wave as illustrated.

A row of overlapping curls is then made, following the half-wave.

That part of the hair which is made into curls should be shaped quite short so it will fluff and flare into place, as shown in the sketch below.

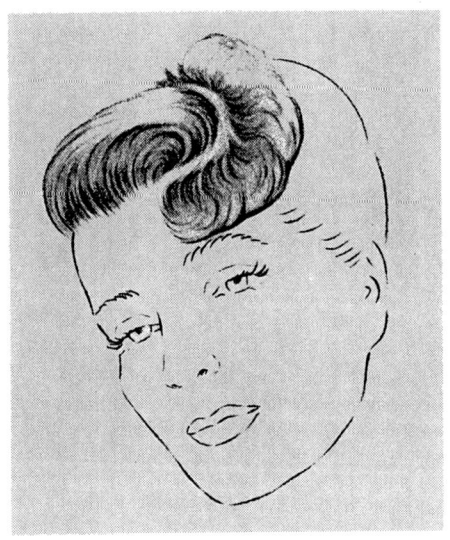

FIGURE 117.

FRENCH BANGS (combed out)

The top hair is combed out in the same direction as it was set—back, and then swirled forward.

To make the curls fluff, lift the comb away from the head as you comb the ends of the hair.

FIGURE 118.

6. FRINGE BANGS

   (setting instructions)

Fringe bangs are the easiest of all to do. A one-half inch wide section of front top hair is cut two inches in length, and set in overlapping forward curls.

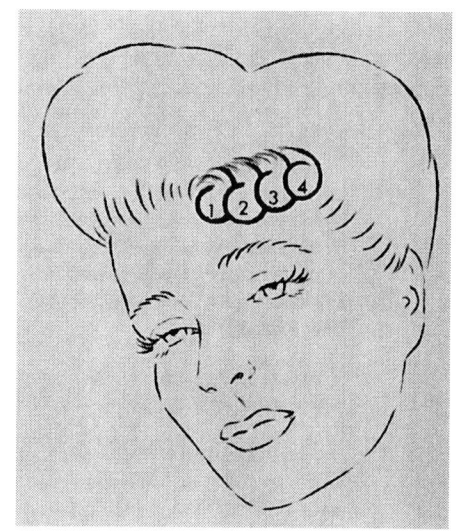

FIGURE 119.

FRINGE BANGS (combed out)

All you need do is run a comb through the hair and allow the short hair to fall as it will. The more careless fringe bangs are, the better.

This sketch shows HALF-FRINGE BANGS. If the bangs extended all the way across the forehead, similiar to the way Bette Davis wore her hair a few years ago, the detail would be called COMPLETE FRINGE BANGS.

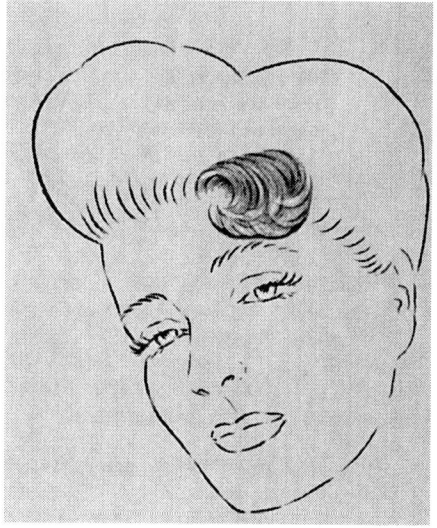

COMBING HINTS

Much of the success of a hairdress depends upon how the various details are combed. The suggestions given here have proved to be of great help to both the hairstylist and the patron.

1. If the hairdress has been set properly and completely dried, it can and should be thoroughly brushed and combed before the final arrangement of the hair. Brushing makes the hairdress appear natural looking and takes away that "I-just-came-from-the-beauty-shop-look." You would be surprised at the great number of women who hurry from a beauty salon to the nearest ladies' lounge so they can really give their hair a good combing. So don't be afraid to vigorously brush your hairstyles.

2. Whenever you have rolls, pomps or bangs, it is usually advisable to comb and brush each detail separately so the partings will not be lost.

3. If the hairdress has curls or fluff on the neck, try combing a little of the crown and nape hair forward towards both ears. "Borrowing" some of the crown and nape hair in this manner gives fullness behind the ears and gives the hair a more pleasing distribution on the head. Following this suggestion will also prevent the hair from buckling in the crown area.

4. When loose curls or a fluff is desired, comb through the curls and lift the comb AWAY from the head. If the hair has been properly shaped, the hair will automatically fall into place.

5. When the nape hair is to be fluffed you can get a beautiful head shape by following this suggestion: comb the crown and nape hair as close to the head as possible. Then firmly press the palm of one hand against the back of the head, and with the comb in the other hand, lift the curls abruptly away from the head. Properly shaped hair will flare into a beautiful cascade of fluff, and the shape of the head in back will be emphasized.

6. When designing a hairstyle take into consideration how capable the patron is at combing her own hair. A beautiful hairstyle is usually not worthwhile if the patron distorts the line the first time she combs it. Your reputation as a hairstylist will be better if you design everyday hairdresses along simple lines so the wearer can comb it satisfactorily herself.

7. All the Six Basic Haircuts are easy to comb because the hair is cut and shaped to fall naturally into place.

8. Hairdressing pomades recondition the hair, give sheen, and a finished look to the hairdress. DO NOT use too much as it will cause the hair to separate and have a "plastered down" look. It is usually a good idea not to use pomades on fine hair.

9. Lacquer can cause the hair to break off when used lavishly by amateurs.

10. This is the most successful way to apply lacquer: first, spray a little lacquer only on the hair nearest the scalp and then comb through the detail to make it smooth. Secondly, spray a thin layer of lacquer over the entire detail and smooth out the drops with the tail end of a tail comb.

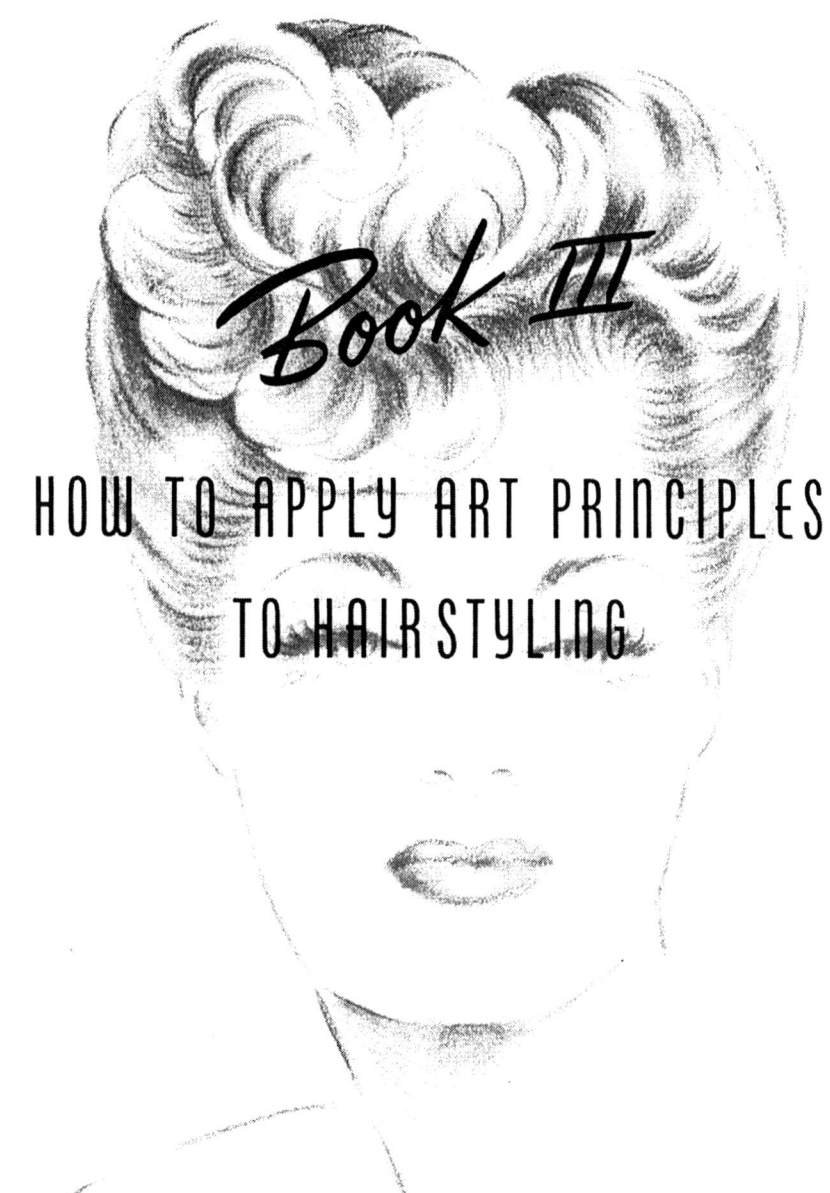

Book III

HOW TO APPLY ART PRINCIPLES TO HAIRSTYLING

THE *Value* OF *Art* IN HAIRSTYLING...

In Book I, we learned the Six Basic Haircuts; in Book II, the Basic Details of Hairstyling. But haircutting and hairstyling is more than a basic or mechanical profession—IT IS AN ART! The true hairstylist must not only know the technical work, but he must also know how to apply art principles to hairshaping and hairstyling. This point can best be illustrated by an analogy.

What is a fifty-dollar hat? Have you ever asked yourself this question? I have, many times. Whenever I heard my patrons raving about the "marvelous fifty-dollar hats they purchased at Saks or John-Frederics," I wondered how a hat could possibly be worth such a price. After all, there is only so much material and so much sewing you can put into a little hat. But after considerable thought, I think I know the answer. The person who designed those fifty-dollar hats had a basic technical knowledge of millinery, and in addition, he knew how to apply art principles in such a way that his hats DO SOMETHING for the women who buy them.

If the hairstyling profession is to be lifted above assembly line hairdresses and hopes to avoid sinking back to cheap prices, we too must learn how to apply art principles in our work. One way to obtain this knowledge is to attend a good art school for two or three years, but most of you have this legitimate excuse: "I don't have the time or money to spend years studying in an art school, and besides I'm not a natural-born artist, so I wouldn't get anything out of the course anyway."

To overcome this problem, the author has narrowed the entire field of art down to a simple, workable basis as it applies to hairstyling, and has drawn sketches to illustrate each point. It is called THE CORRECT MASS OUTLINE METHOD OF HAIRSTYLING. This method applies to all types of hairdresses, and even though you are not a natural-born artist, it will make it possible for you to know WHY most hairdresses are unbecoming and HOW to make them becoming.

THE CORRECT MASS OUTLINE METHOD OF HAIRSTYLING is not theoretical—it is as fundamentally sound as art itself, and will teach you how to develop good taste and a flawless hairstyling technique. The Correct Mass Outline Method of Hairstyling has been used successfully by the author in hairstyling contests and in the beauty salon for years.

Directors of Beauty Culture Schools can do much to enhance their reputations for turning out ultra-competent hairstylists by including The Correct Mass Outline Method of Hairstyling in their curricula, for their graduates will be able to walk into any salon and quickly prove their styling ability.

THE CORRECT *Mass Outline Method* OF HAIRSTYLING

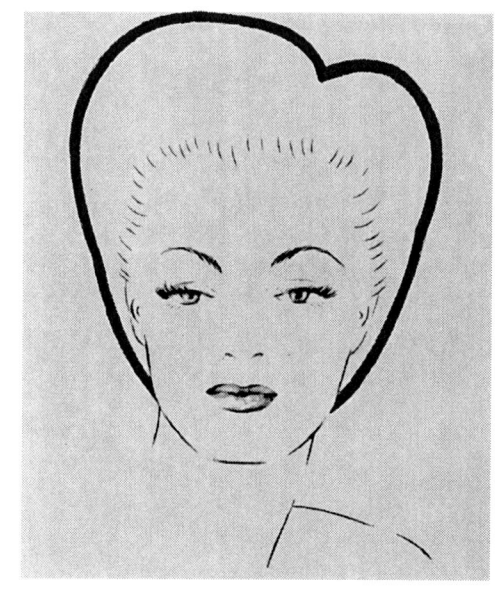

FIGURE 120.

MASS OUTLINE is defined as the outside border of a hairdress as shown by the heavy lines in this sketch.

Throughout Book III, the heavy lines in the sketches will indicate the mass outline of the hairdress.

THE CORRECT MASS OUTLINE METHOD OF HAIRSTYLING will be studied in these five phases:

1. The Correct Mass Outline must have good balance.

2. From a front view, The Correct Mass Outline Method of Hairstyling teaches how to determine the most becoming hairstyle lines.

3. From a side view, The Correct Mass Outline Method of Hairstyling teaches how to determine the most becoming hairstyle lines.

4. The Correct Mass Outline Method of Hairstyling teaches how to arrange hair to overcome facial and head irregularities.

5. The Correct Mass Outline Method of Hairstyling teaches how to design the most becoming hairstyles for the five face types.

1. THE CORRECT MASS OUTLINE MUST HAVE GOOD BALANCE...

The correct mass outline of a hairdress must, first of all, have good balance. One good way to learn balance is to get in the habit of asking yourself this question, "Is the mass outline of the hairdress pleasing?"

There are two kinds of balance in hairdressing: Center Balance, and Off-Center Balance.

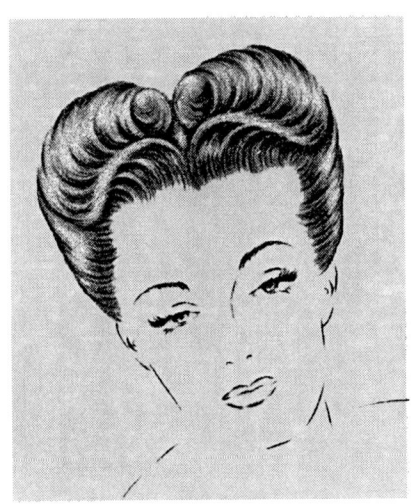

FIGURE 121. CENTER BALANCE

When both sides of the center are arranged exactly the same, the hairdress has center balance. An example is the hairdress in this sketch which has identical hair arrangements on both sides.

It is also possible to have center balance when no part shows from a front view. An example is a straight back pompadour.

Center balance has a tendency to be monotonous and is becoming to very few women.

FIGURE 122. OFF-CENTER BALANCE

A hairdress has off-center balance when both sides of the center are not exactly the same, but the hairdress as a whole *appears* to be balanced because both sides attract equal attention.

Off-center balance is more artistic, more becoming, and makes possible a greater variety of designs than does center balance.

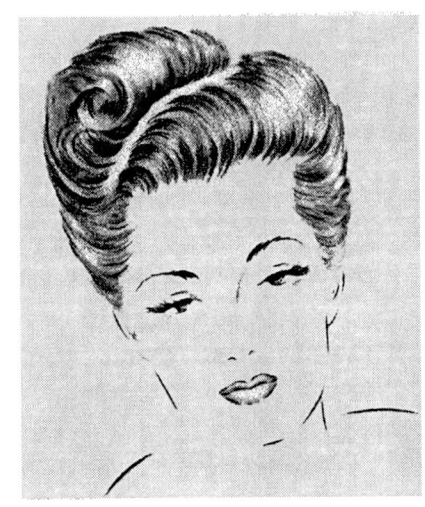

FIGURE 123.
AN UNBALANCED HAIRDRESS

Look at this sketch and ask yourself this question, "Is the mass outline of the hairdress pleasing?"

Your answer should be "no," because the mass outline has a disturbing effect, and one wonders what keeps the top-heavy hair arrangement up and how soon it will fall down.

As you study the remaining pages of this Volume you will gradually acquire the ability to design hairstyles with perfect balance.

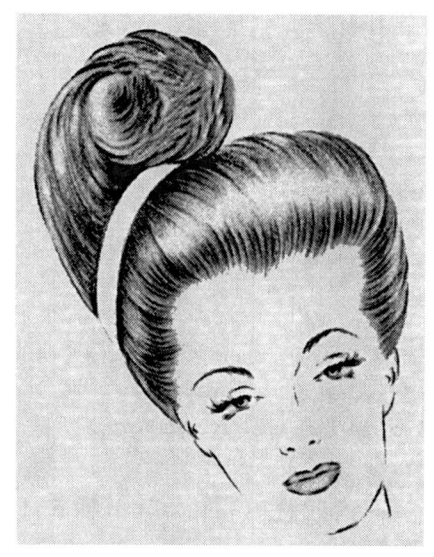

2. FROM A FRONT VIEW, THE CORRECT MASS OUTLINE METHOD OF HAIRSTYLING TEACHES HOW TO DETERMINE THE MOST BECOMING HAIRSTYLE LINES...

This phase of The Correct Mass Outline Method of Hairstyling is based primarily on the artistic premise that the oval face is ideal, and that curved lines are more becoming than straight lines.

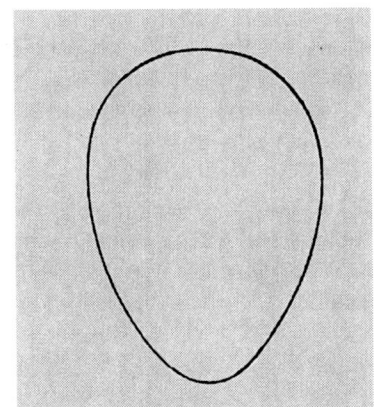

FIGURE 124. This drawing shows the ideal oval. It is shaped like an egg standing upright on the small end.

Since the application of the oval shape is essential to successful hairstyling, it is suggested that you study and memorize this oval shape.

Today our leading illustrators favor models with oval faces; studio make-up artists apply the tricks of their trade to make the star's face appear oval, and the millinery experts design hats that make the wearer's face look oval.

It is reasonable then, since the oval face is considered ideal, to design the mass outline of the hairstyle in such a way that a natural oval face will remain oval-looking, and if the face is not oval, the mass outline of the hair should be designed to make it appear more oval in shape than it actually is.

The mass outlines of all hairdresses are divided into these four groups when seen from a direct front view:

      (a) hair visible from the ears up.
      (b) hair visible from the chin-line up.
      (c) all down lines.
      (d) combination of high and low lines.

Now we will illustrate incorrect and correct mass outlines for each of these four groups.

IF THE HAIR IS VISIBLE ONLY FROM THE EARS UP

FIGURE 125. INCORRECT MASS OUTLINE:

The mass outline of the hair, plus the outline of the lower half of the face, does not have a general oval shape.

(By "general oval shape," I do not mean perfectly oval, as in Figure 124. The mass outline of a hairdress may be irregular in shape, but still have an approximate, or general oval shape.)

The hair is flat on top, and too wide at the sides.

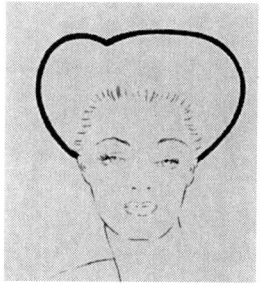

FIGURE 126. CORRECT MASS OUTLINE:

The mass outline of the hair, plus the outline of the lower half of the face, has a general oval shape as illustrated.

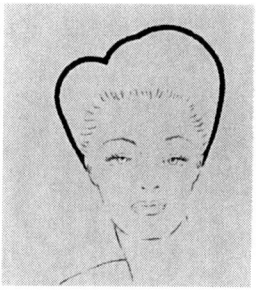

IF THE HAIR IS VISIBLE ONLY FROM THE CHIN LINE UP

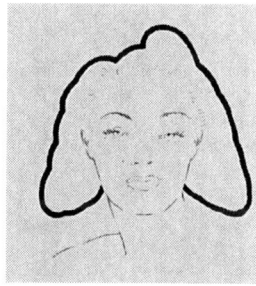

FIGURE 127. INCORRECT MASS OUTLINE:

The mass outline of the hair, plus the chin line, does not have a general oval shape.

The hair arrangement is too wide at the bottom and too narrow at the temples.

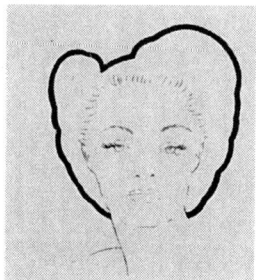

FIGURE 128. CORRECT MASS OUTLINE:

The mass outline of the hair, plus the chin line, has a general oval shape.

This correct mass outline is particularly good for Baby and Middy Haircuts when the hair is brushed out in loose fluff at the sides and neck.

IF ALL THE HAIR HAS A DOWN LINE, AND FALLS IN LOOSE CURLS ON THE NECK

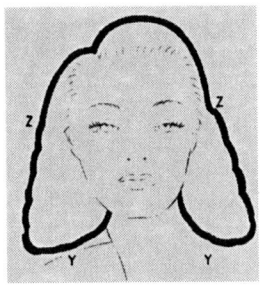

FIGURE 129. INCORRECT MASS OUTLINE:

The hair arrangement is too narrow from the temples up.

The loose curls on the neck have poor mass outline, because the hair at "Y" is not longest, and the outline of the curls from "Y" to "Z" does not have a crescent curve.

(Crescent Curve is defined as "The shape of the visible part of the moon in its first or last quarter.")

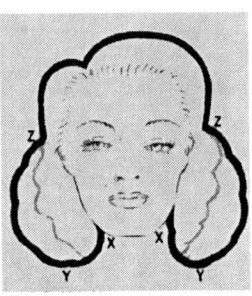

FIGURE 130. CORRECT MASS OUTLINE:

The mass outline of the hair, (excluding the curls from "Z" to "X"), plus the outline of the lower half of the face, has a general oval shape.

The hair is longest at "Y" and gradually gets shorter toward "X".

The mass outline of the curls from "Y" to "Z" has a crescent curve.

IF THE HAIRDRESS HAS A COMBINATION OF HIGH AND LOW LINES

FIGURE 131. INCORRECT MASS OUTLINE:

The hair is too wide at the temples, and not high enough on top.

The hair at "Y" is not longest.

The outline of the curls from "Y" to "Z" does not take a graceful crescent curve.

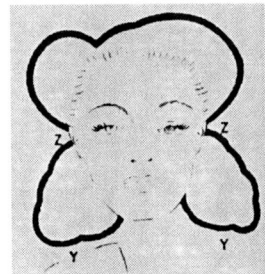

FIGURE 132. CORRECT MASS OUTLINE:

The mass outline of the top and sides, (excluding the curls from "Z" to "X"), plus the outline of the lower half of the face, has a general oval shape.

The hair is longest at "Y" and gradually gets shorter toward "X".

The mass outline of the curls from "Y" to "Z" has a crescent curve.

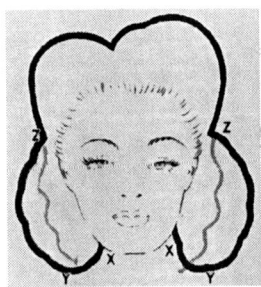

Because there are so many high hair arrangements with rolls at the neck, we will also give incorrect and correct mass outlines to illustrate this type of high-low combination hairdress.

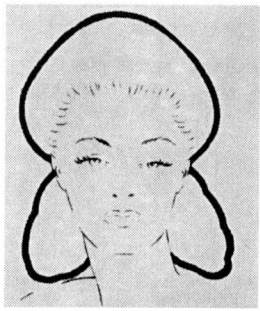

FIGURE 133. INCORRECT MASS OUTLINE:

The hair arrangement comes to a point at the top.

The roll on the neck does not have a crescent curve outline.

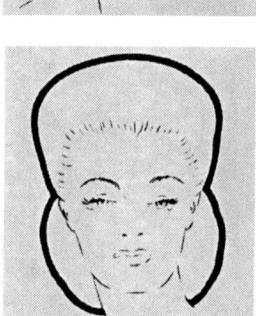

FIGURE 134. CORRECT MASS OUTLINE:

The mass outline of the top and sides, (excluding the roll on the neck), plus the outline of the lower half of the face, has a general oval shape.

The roll in back has a crescent curve outline.

3. FROM A SIDE VIEW, THE CORRECT MASS OUTLINE METHOD OF HAIRSTYLING TEACHES HOW TO DETERMINE THE MOST BECOMING HAIRSTYLE LINES...

This phase of The Correct Mass Outline Method of Hairstyling is based primarily on the following art principles: harmony, proportion, balance, rhythm, and crescent curves.

IF A HAIRDRESS IS BEING DESIGNED FOR A SHINGLE HAIRCUT

FIGURE 135.
INCORRECT MASS OUTLINE:

The mass outline of this hair arrangement gives the head a severe mannish look.

Top hair is flat and uninteresting.

The lower nape hair was clipped too close to the head.

There are unforgivable step-offs because the nape and crown hair was not shaped properly.

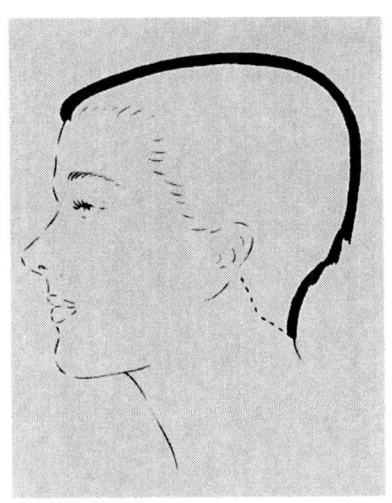

FIGURE 136.
CORRECT MASS OUTLINE:

The mass outline of the hair gives a soft, feminine shape to the head.

The top hair is arranged in an irregular mass outline with limited height.

The lower nape hair is full enough to make the base of the skull appear to have a pleasing roundness.

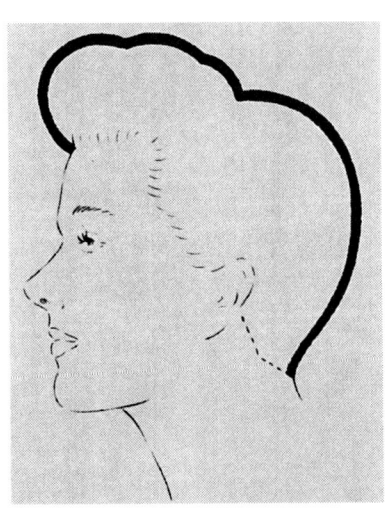

IF THE HAIR IS LONG AND THE HAIRDRESS HAS AN ALL UP LINE

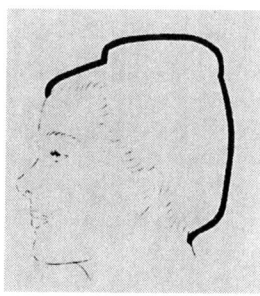

FIGURE 137. INCORRECT MASS OUTLINE:

The hair detail on the top extends too far back and distorts the beautiful curved formation of the crown.

♦ The straight up-and-down line makes the back of the head appear flat.

The bulge at the base of the skull also distorts the shape of the head.

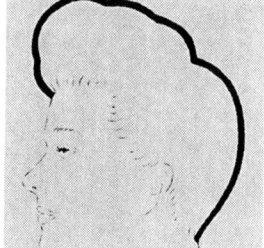

FIGURE 138. CORRECT MASS OUTLINE

♦ The roll, or fluff effect on top is placed well to the front and does not extend too far back into the crown area.

The nape hair is arranged close to the head and gives a pleasing, feminine roundness to the back of the head.

IF THE HAIRDRESS HAS ALL DOWN LINES

FIGURE 139. INCORRECT MASS OUTLINE:

The hair on top is flat and uninteresting.

The hair does not curve in at the base of the skull.

The hair is too short at "Y", and does not gradually ♦ get shorter towards "X".

The outline of the hair from "Y" to "Z" does not have a crescent curve.

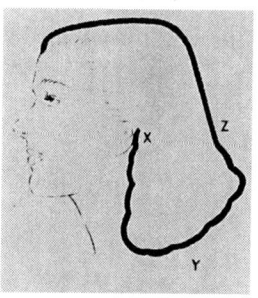

FIGURE 140. CORRECT MASS OUTLINE:

The top hair is slightly higher in the front and has a soft line.

The hair curves in at the base of the skull and shows ♦ the head formation.

The hair is longest at "Y", and gradually gets shorter towards "X."

The fluff from "Y" to "Z" has a crescent curve outline.

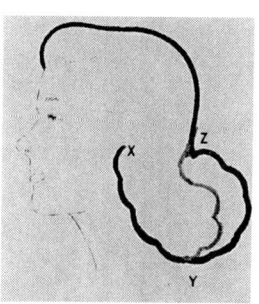

IF THE HAIRDRESS HAS A COMBINATION OF HIGH AND LOW LINES

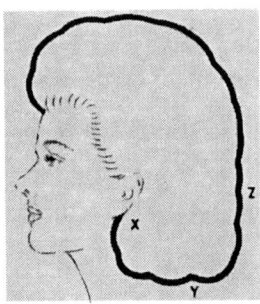

FIGURE 141. INCORRECT MASS OUTLINE:

The top hair arrangement continues into the crown area.

The fluff on the neck does not flare abruptly away from the base of the skull, so the round formation of the back of the head has been lost.

The hair does not gradually get shorter from "Y" to "X."

The curls on the neck from "Y" to "Z" do not have a crescent curve outline.

All in all, this fussy, overloaded hairdress suggests inferior workmanship and poor taste.

Another common incorrect mass outline for a combination high and low hairdress is illustrated in this sketch.

FIGURE 142. INCORRECT MASS OUTLINE:

The hair arrangement on the top of the head extends too far into the crown area.

The line from "A" to "Z" is straight, and so does not show the formation of the head.

The outline of the curls from "Y" to "Z" does not have a crescent curve.

The hair does not gradually get shorter from "Y" to "X."

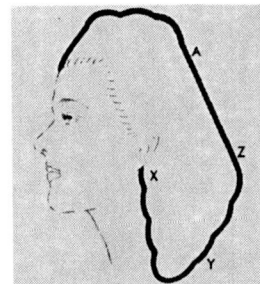

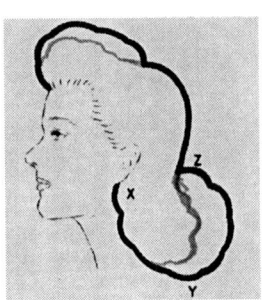

FIGURE 143. CORRECT MASS OUTLINE:

The top hair arrangement is kept to the front of the head, and does not extend too far into the crown area.

The fluff on the neck flares abruptly away from the base of the skull. This gives a pleasing shape to the back of the head.

The hair on the neck is longest at "Y", and gradually gets shorter toward "X."

The curls from "Y" to "Z" have a crescent curve outline.

4. THE CORRECT MASS OUTLINE METHOD OF HAIRSTYLING TEACHES HOW TO ARRANGE HAIR TO OVERCOME FACIAL AND HEAD IRREGULARITIES...

This phase of The Correct Mass Outline Method of Hairstyling is based primarily on the following art principles:

    (a) Round lines are more becoming than straight lines.
    (b) Lines which take the same direction emphasize each other.
    (c) Proportion, balance, rhythm, and harmony.
    (d) Concealment. Whenever an abnormality such as scars or large ears cannot be made to appear normal by optical illusion, the irregularity may sometimes be concealed by arranging the hair to cover it.

IF THE HEAD IS FLAT ON TOP

FIGURE 144. INCORRECT MASS OUTLINE:

The mass outline of the top hair is low and flat.

The horizontal line of the top hair repeats the line of the top of the head, and thus the flatness of the head is emphasized.

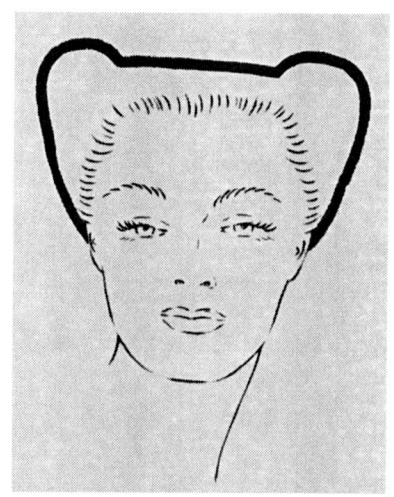

FIGURE 145. CORRECT MASS OUTLINE:

The top hair arrangement is high, and has an irregular mass outline.

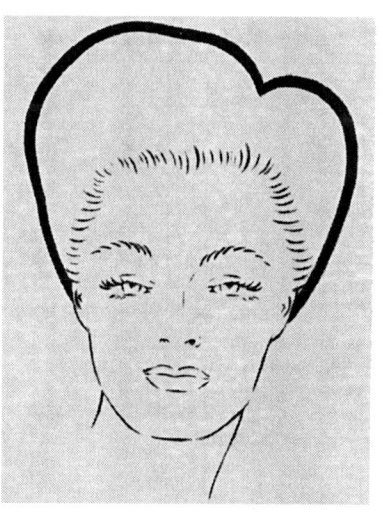

IF THE UPPER HALF OF THE FACE IS LONG (High Forehead)

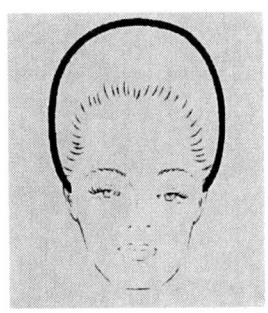

FIGURE 146. INCORRECT MASS OUTLINE:

The high forehead is exposed.

◀ The longness of the upper half of the face is emphasized by the high hair arrangement.

The hairdress is narrow, and thus makes the upper half of the face look longer.

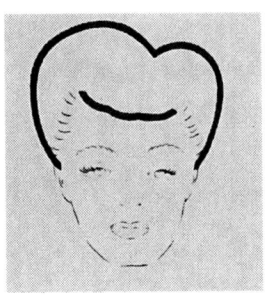

FIGURE 147. CORRECT MASS OUTLINE:

◀ The bangs and limited height of the hairdress make the forehead appear normal.

IF THE UPPER HALF OF THE FACE IS SHORT (Low Forehead)

FIGURE 148. INCORRECT MASS OUTLINE:

The hair arrangement is flat on top.   ▶

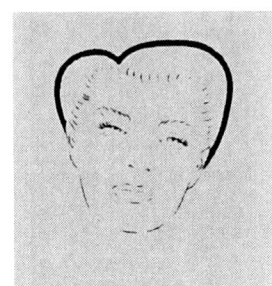

FIGURE 149. CORRECT MASS OUTLINE:

The hair has a high, irregular mass outline that causes the upper half of the face to appear longer and in good proportion.   ▶

Bangs may sometimes be used to advantage if the style has height.

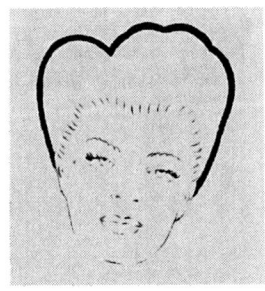

IF THE TEMPLES ARE NARROW

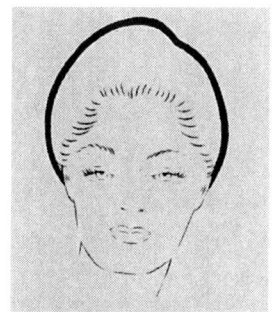

FIGURE 150. INCORRECT MASS OUTLINE:

Because the hair converges to a point on top, the narrowness of the temples is emphasized.

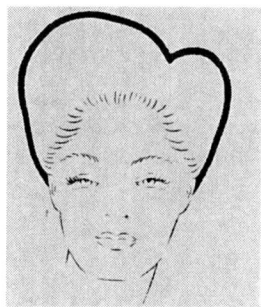

FIGURE 151. CORRECT MASS OUTLINE:

The mass outline of the hair from the ears up, plus the outline of the lower half of the face, has a general oval shape.

IF THE NOSE IS CROOKED

FIGURE 152. INCORRECT MASS OUTLINE:

The center balance and center part divide the head in two equal parts, and thus cause the nose to be even more conspicuous.

Notice the dotted line in this sketch. If the part were here, the crooked nose would also be emphasized, because the part would take the same direction as the nose.

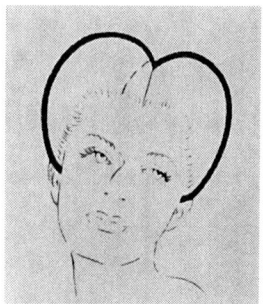

FIGURE 153. CORRECT MASS OUTLINE:

Hair arrangement has a soft irregular mass outline.

The off-center balance attracts the eye away from the nose.

(Side parts are good if they do not repeat the line of the crooked nose.)

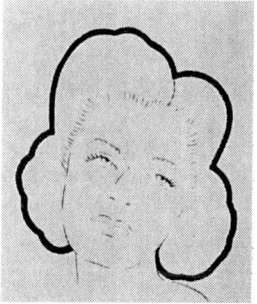

IF THE NOSE IS LONG

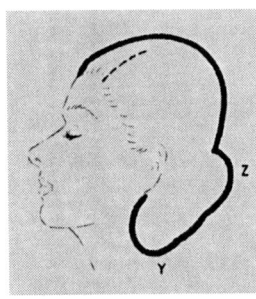

FIGURE 154. INCORRECT MASS OUTLINE:

The top hair continues approximately the same line as the nose, and for this reason emphasizes the length of the nose.

The hair arrangement on the neck from "Y" to "Z" is too harsh, and repeats the line of the nose.

The up-diagonal part is bad, because it takes the same direction as the nose.

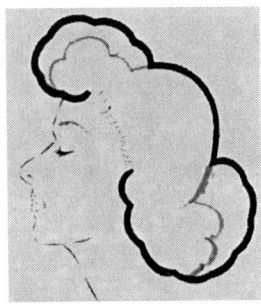

FIGURE 155. CORRECT MASS OUTLINE:

The top hair is well to the front, and has a soft mass outline. This draws the eye away from the nose, and gives better proportion to the upper half of the face.

The hair on the neck and over the ears is full and casual.

IF THE EARS ARE LARGE OR DEFORMED

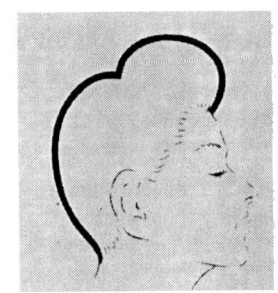

FIGURE 156. INCORRECT MASS OUTLINE:

The ears are entirely exposed.

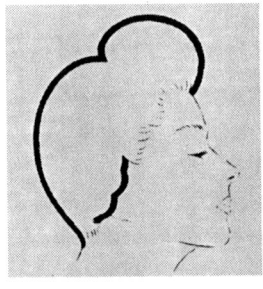

FIGURE 157. CORRECT MASS OUTLINE:

By applying the art principle of concealment, a soft hair arrangement is designed to cover all but the ear lobes.

IF THE CHIN RECEDES

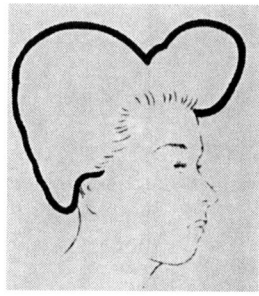

FIGURE 158. INCORRECT MASS OUTLINE:

◀ The mass outline of the hair is too wide at the top, and because it narrows down, the eye is attracted to the receding chin.

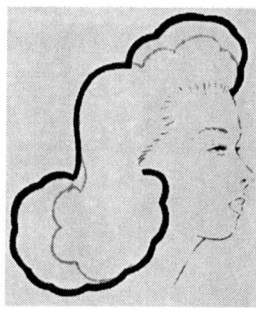

FIGURE 159. CORRECT MASS OUTLINE:

The top hair is full, and is irregular in shape.

◀ The soft hair arrangement on the neck and over the ears gives good proportion to the lower half of the face, and draws the eye away from the receding chin.

These incorrect and correct mass outlines also apply to a PROTRUDING JAW.

IF THE NECK IS LONG

FIGURE 160. INCORRECT MASS OUTLINE:

The hairdress has an all-up line.

The outline of the hair at the sides is almost straight ◀ up and down. These vertical lines take the same direction as the neck lines, and make the neck appear longer and thinner than it really is.

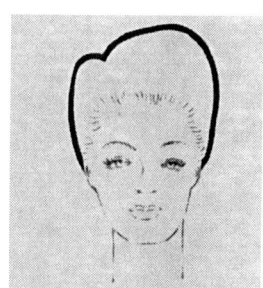

FIGURE 161. CORRECT MASS OUTLINE:

The haircut may be either a Middy Plus or Long ◀ length.

The hair arrangement at the neck is soft and casual.

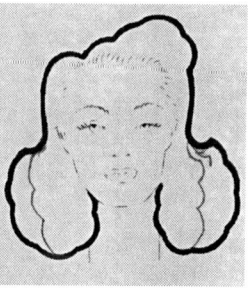

IF THE FOREHEAD RECEDES

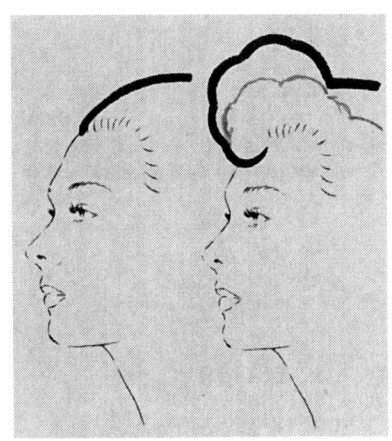

FIGURE 162.
INCORRECT MASS OUTLINE:

The top hair continues the line of the receding forehead, thus emphasizing the bad feature.

CORRECT MASS OUTLINE:

The soft bangs conceal the upper haif of the forehead and make it appear normal.

5. THE CORRECT MASS OUTLINE METHOD OF HAIRSTYLING TEACHES HOW TO DESIGN THE MOST BECOMING HAIRSTYLES FOR THE FIVE FACE TYPES...

From the hairstylist's point of view, faces are best classified as being OVAL, ROUND, SQUARE, LONG, and HEART. After you have learned how to style hair for these five face types, you will then be prepared to successfully design hairstyles for all face types or combinations of face types.

When analyzing a patron's face to determine the shape of her face, first look at the chin—it will usually give you the clue.

If her chin is:

(a) shaped like the lower part of an egg, she may have an oval face.
(b) round, her face in most cases will be round.
(c) square, her face is probably square.
(d) long and narrow, her face is usually long.
(e) pointed, her face is probably heart shaped.

Remember, these hairstyling suggestions for face types are not hard and fast rules—they will not apply to all faces because all faces do not fall into one of the five categories. Most faces are a combination of different types. The following mass outline suggestions will provide a background that will be invaluable for designing hairstyles for any face because they are basic art principles.

OVAL FACE

If your face is this type you are extremely lucky—almost any hairstyle you choose will be becoming, provided the mass outline has good balance and is in proper proportion.

PROBLEM: To keep the face oval-looking.

FIGURE 163. INCORRECT MASS OUTLINE:

Too bad! Our perfect face has been distorted by incorrect mass outline.

"A" to "B" is flat.
"C" to "D" is vertical.
"D" to "E" does not have a crescent curve.

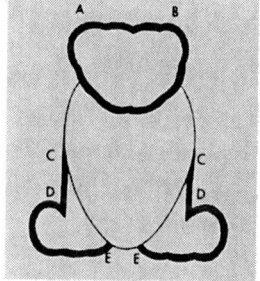

FIGURE 164. CORRECT MASS OUTLINE:

The mass outline of the top and sides, (excluding the curls from "D" to "E"), plus the outline of the lower half of the face, has a general oval shape.

The outline of the curls from "D" to "E" has a crescent curve.

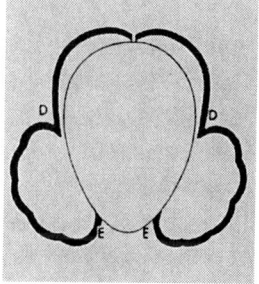

IF THE FACE IS ROUND

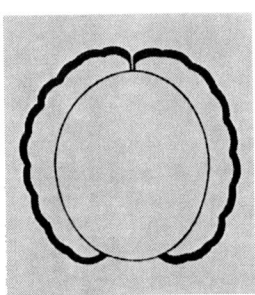

PROBLEM: To design a hairdress that will make the face appear longer.

FIGURE 165. INCORRECT MASS OUTLINE:

The center part and center balance seem to divide the face in two equal parts, and this emphasizes the roundness of the face.

The mass outline of the hair repeats the round line of the face.

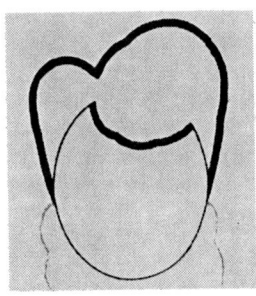

FIGURE 166. CORRECT MASS OUTLINE:

High, irregular hair arrangement on top.

Sides close to the head.

Soft bangs break up the round lines of the face.

IF THE FACE IS SQUARE

PROBLEM: To design a hairdress that will lengthen and give roundness to the face.

FIGURE 167. INCORRECT MASS OUTLINE:

The center part seems to divide the face in half and emphasizes its squareness.

The mass outline of the hair repeats the square lines of the face.

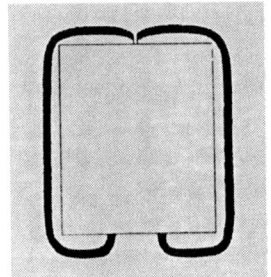

FIGURE 168. CORRECT MASS OUTLINE:

Rounded side part.

High, irregular mass outline.

The mass outline of the hair at the sides of the head takes a graceful curve, and gives the face an illusion of roundness.

Soft bangs with crescent curve. (By all means do not use bangs that have straight lines.)

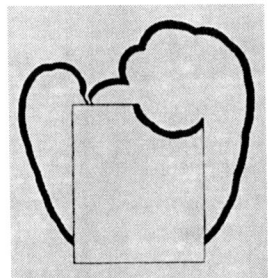

IF THE FACE IS LONG

PROBLEM: To design a hairdress that will make the face appear shorter and more round.

FIGURE 169. INCORRECT MASS OUTLINE:

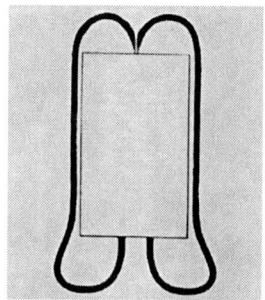

Center part, and center balance, make the face appear longer than it really is.

Too much height on top.

Side hair too close to the head.

Long, droopy hair on the neck does not have a crescent curve.

FIGURE 170. CORRECT MASS OUTLINE:

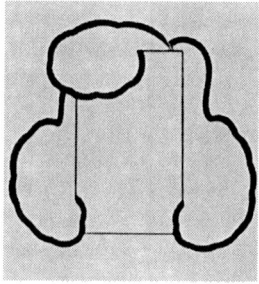

Up diagonal part gives width to the top of the head, and allows more hair to fall on the small side. This extra hair on the small side is needed for fullness on the neck.

French bangs break up the long line of the face and give an illusion of width.

Fullness at the sides makes the face appear more round.

Low, soft curls, or fluff, cause the long face to be less noticeable.

IF THE FACE IS HEART SHAPE

Most make-up artists classify this type face as the "inverted triangle," but for hairstyling purposes it is more convenient to call it "heart shape."

PROBLEM: To design a hairdress that will make the lower half of the face appear fuller, and give an illusion of roundness to the top of the head.

FIGURE 171. INCORRECT MASS OUTLINE:

Center part seems to divide the head in half and thus focus attention on the pointed chin.

Hair is flat on top and too wide at the temples.

The mass outline of the entire hairdress repeats the heart shape of the face.

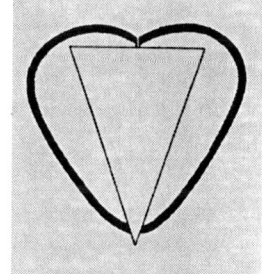

FIGURE 172. CORRECT MASS OUTLINE:

Side part and off-center balance detract attention from the pointed chin.

High, irregular mass outline on the top of head gives an illusion of roundness.

Loose curls cause the lower half of the face to appear fuller.

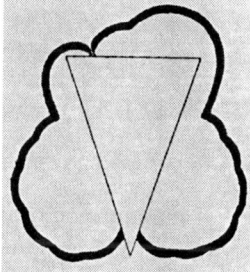

GENERAL ART RULES FOR HAIRSTYLING

1. Properly shaped and tapered hair is more flattering than hair which is all the same length.

2. Loose, fluffy curls are more becoming than small, tight curls.

3. Wide, soft waves are more artistic and flattering than narrow, ridgy waves.

4. Up-lines in a hairdress make one appear buoyant, and seem to erase facial lines. If your patron has the features to wear an all-up coiffure, design one for her sometime and she will be surprised to find how it lifts her spirits and swings her into the mood for a gay evening.

5. Down-lines in a hair arrangement accentuate a double chin and facial lines.

6. Scars and deep wrinkles on the forehead can be hidden by bangs. If there are wens or bumps on the head, decide on a part that does not show them and arrange the hair in rolls or bangs to cover them. If there are scars or birth marks behind the ears, plan fullness so the defect will be concealed.

7. If glasses are worn, the top hair should be arranged in loose, irregular lines.

8. The shape of the face will be emphasized if the hairdress follows the same lines. For example, a square face appears even more square when the style is flat on top and has straight up-and-down lines at the sides.

9. Center parts are not advisable when there is a definite widow's peak.

10. Small faces are best complimented by a style that is soft, wispy, and in proportion to the size of the head. Excessively large or small hairdresses should be avoided.

11. Women with large faces should wear wide waves and full rolls. Fussy details are out.

12. The problem of a short neck is best solved by wearing the hair high with the ears partly showing. This gives an illusion of a longer neck. A swirled back with diagonal waves is suitable.

13. Sloping shoulders are best counteracted by a style that is low and full on the neck. Avoid hairdresses that have all-up lines.

14. Broad shoulders are emphasized when the lines of a hairdress are horizontal.

15. Short women can add inches to their height by wearing high hairdresses.

16. Tall women should not emphasize their height by wearing high hairdresses. The hair should be kept quite flat on top with fullness at the sides.

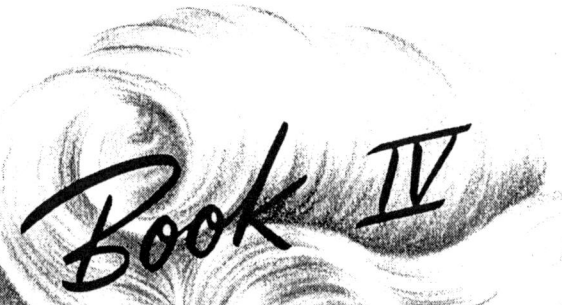

Book IV

HOW TO DESIGN HAIRSTYLES SO THEY WILL BE SUITABLE TO PERSONALITY, AGE, AND OCCASION

All the hairstyles in Book IV are made possible by the application of the Hairshaping and Hairstyling Methods explained in this Volume.

In the first three Books, we learned The Guide Method of Haircutting, The Basic Details of Hairstyling, and The Correct Mass Outline Method of Hairstyling. But in addition, the master hairstylist must know which hairstyles are suitable to:

    The Patron's personality

    The Patron's age

    The occasion on which they are to be worn.

THE HAIRSTYLE MUST BE SUITABLE TO THE PATRON'S PERSONALITY..

It is quite possible for two women to have identical figures, and the same type of face and hair, but still have totally different personalities. To illustrate this point, suppose one of these patrons is a University Dean of Women, and the other is Mazie, the gum-chewing, boisterous, hash-slinger at Joe's Beanery. Would you give them the same hairdress? Obviously not. The Dean of Women would be very uncomfortable wearing Mazie's long, fluffy, bleached hairdress—and Mazie's gum would probably take a worse beating if she had to wear the Dean's conservative coiffure.

The key then, to designing a hairdress that is suitable to personality is this: women who have quiet, dignified, reserved personalities usually should have conservative hairstyles—while the extrovert, who strives to be the center of attention, loves to have her hair arranged in eye-catching styles.

THE HAIRSTYLE MUST BE SUITABLE TO THE PATRON'S AGE...

There are no hard and fast rules that we can follow to help us to determine which hairstyles should be worn by women in the different age groups. During my career as a stylist, I can recall several instances when the same hairstyle looked equally well when worn by both the mother and her twenty-year-old daughter. For this reason, I wish to make it clear that the suggested hairstyles in this book may, in some cases, be worn to advantage by women of other age groups.

1. HAIRSTYLES FOR THE "JUNIOR MISS"

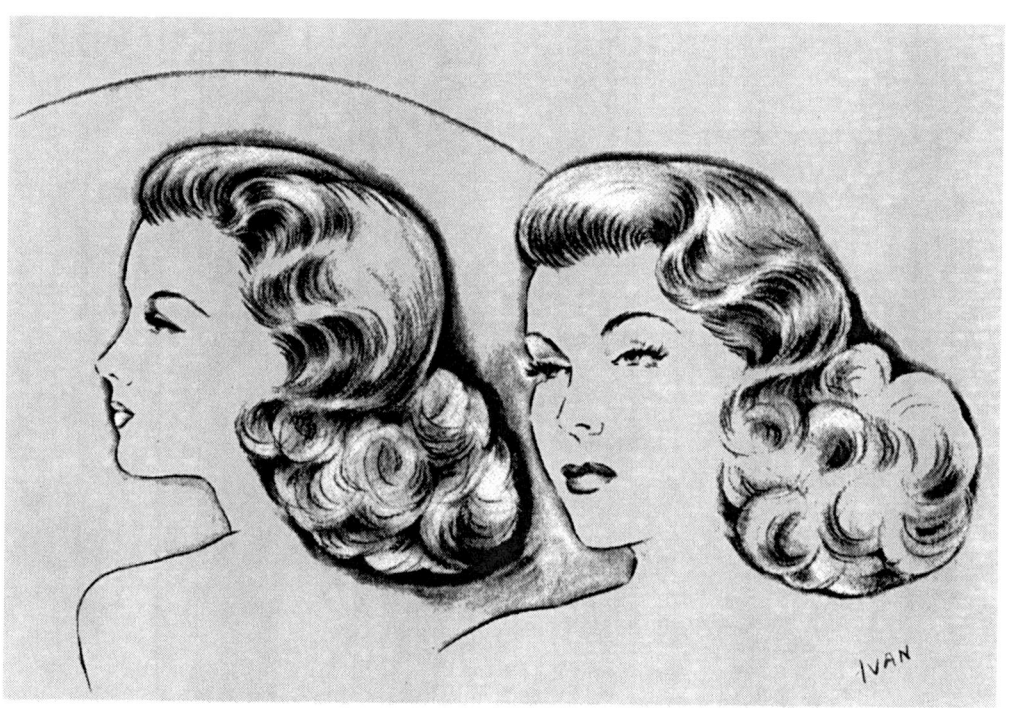

FIGURE 173. MIDDY PLUS HAIRCUT

DETAILS: Wide waves, and fluff.

REMARKS:

- (a) When setting the large side, comb the top hair almost straight back before swirling the hair forward to make the waves.

- (b) Notice the small side takes an up, and backward direction near the part.

- (c) Some of the crown and nape hair is combed toward the ears to provide extra fullness.

FIGURE 174. BABY HAIRCUT

DETAILS:

(a) "V" part.

(b) Modified stand-up half-wave plus fluff bangs on top.

(c) Both sides have a wide, vertical wave followed by fluff.

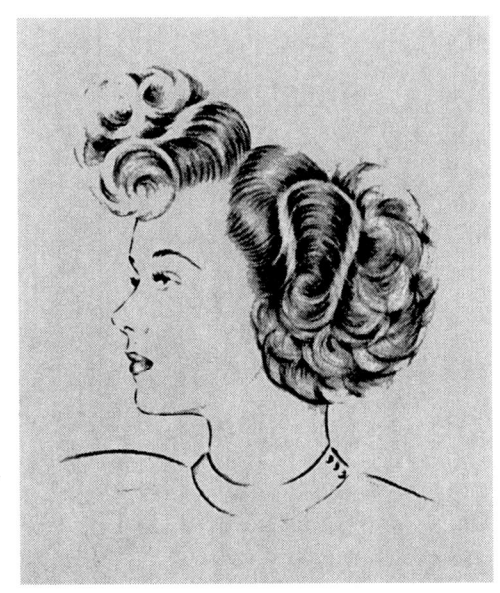

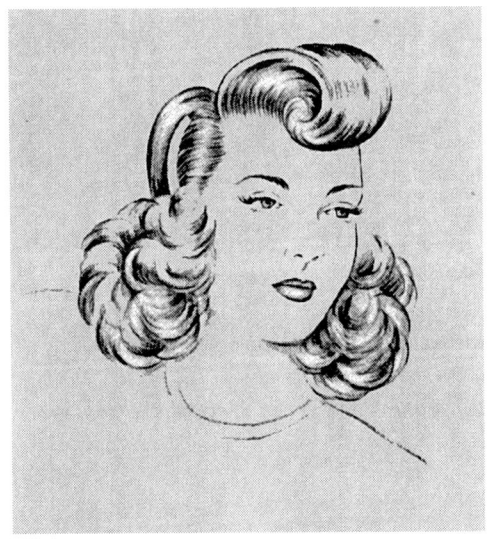

FIGURE 175. MIDDY PLUS HAIRCUT

DETAILS:

(a) "V" part.

(b) Modified forward roll bangs.

(c) Right and left side hair is combed back off the face and held in place by combs.

(d) Fluff at neck and over ears.

2. HAIRSTYLES FOR YOUNG WOMEN

FIGURE 176. LONG HAIRCUT
in combination with—

(a) Top hair is cut to pomp length.

(b) Sides are half-wave reverse roll length.

DETAILS:

(a) Ear-to-ear part.

(b) Combination of pomp on top with up vertical half-wave reverse rolls at the sides.

(c) Fluff at neck and over ears.

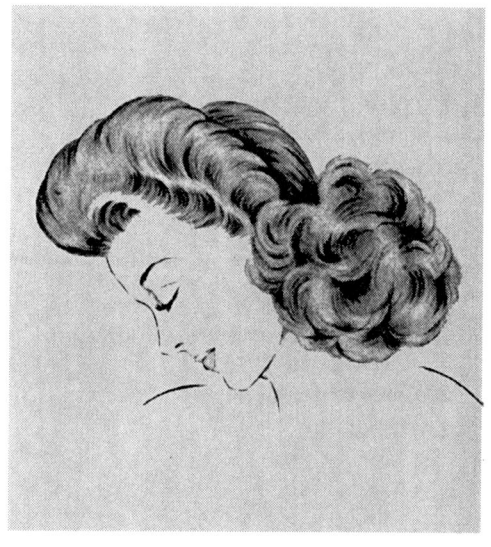

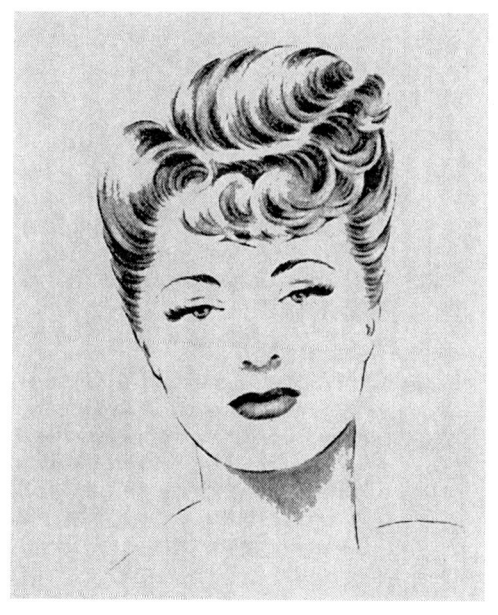

FIGURE 177. MIDDY HAIRCUT
in combination with—

(a) Top hair is cut to half-wave bangs length.

(b) Sides are cut to reverse roll length.

DETAILS:

(a) Ear-to-ear part plus right and left side parts.

(b) Half-wave bangs with soft curls.

(c) Reverse roll on either side.

(d) The back is swirled with a cluster of curls back of the left ear.

REMARKS:

(a) This model has a round face. To give an illusion of length, a rat is inserted under the bangs and the sides are kept close to the head.

FIGURE 178. MIDDY HAIRCUT
in combination with—

(a) Bangs are cut two and one-half inches in length.

DETAILS:
(a) "V" part.
(b) Fluff bangs on top.
(c) Sides have an up vertical half-wave with curls.
(d) Curls on neck and over ears.

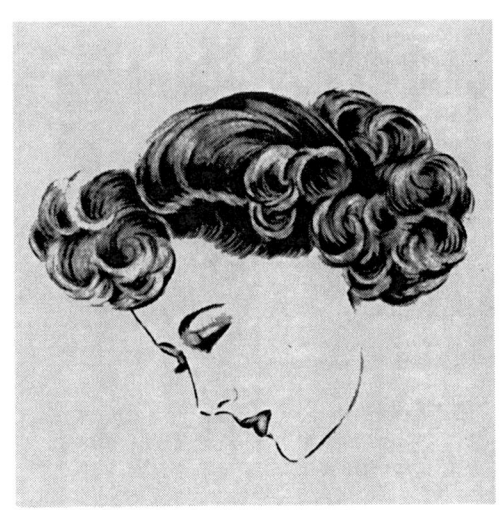

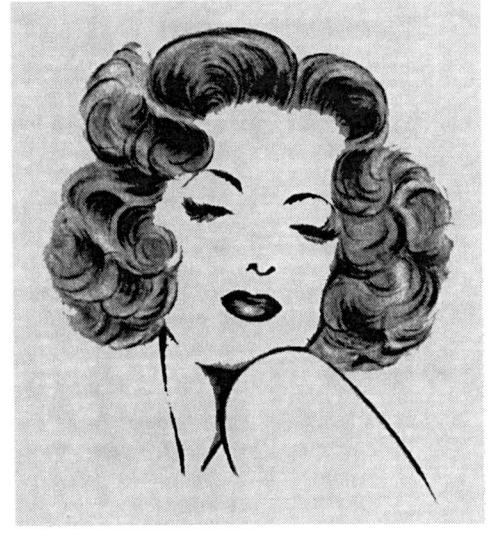

FIGURE 179. MIDDY HAIRCUT

DETAILS:
(a) The small side has a half-wave followed by fluff.
(b) The large side has two complete waves with fluff interspersed.
(c) The back is smooth with fluff on the neck.

REMARKS:
(a) Notice how this Middy Haircut is shaped around the face to eliminate all excessive length and hair weight. Many times a Middy Haircut will bring out natural waves that the patron did not know she possessed.

3. HAIRSTYLES FOR CHIC MATRONS

The dictionary defines the word "matron" as "a middle-aged woman of dignity." The suggested hairstyles for this group were especially designed to enhance that dignity.

Women in this group are pretty well established in life. Their children are off to college or married, and household duties are no longer a full-time job. Naturally, the matron turns to club work and social functions. This new position in life demands that she wear fashionable dresses and hats, and of course, a professional-looking hairstyle.

Our problem then, is to create styles that are smart, becoming, and have simple lines. To accomplish this we will concentrate on wide waves, full rolls, and hair arrangements above the collar. We will avoid tight little curls, and all details that might suggest that she is trying to copy the "glamour-teen."

Matrons are particularly hat conscious and frequently desire to change their hairstyles to "go with" their latest millinery finds. Progressive hairstylists should be on the alert to caution their "hat-happy" patrons that their best hairstyle lines are of primary importance, and that new chapeaux should be purchased *only if they compliment their best hairstyle lines.*

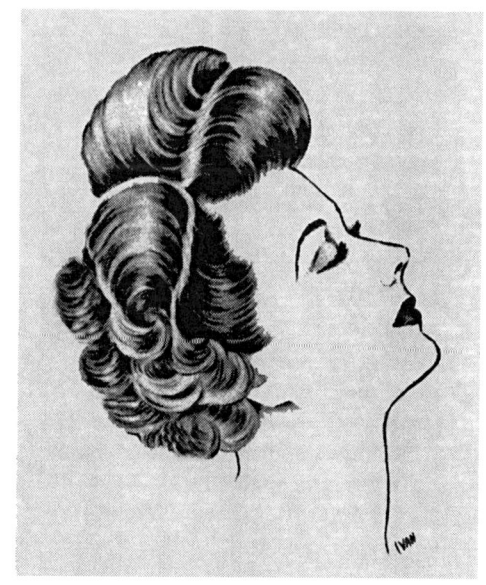

FIGURE 180. BABY HAIRCUT
in combination with—

(a) Top hair is half-wave reverse roll length.

DETAILS:

(a) Rectangular part.
(b) Stand-up half-wave reverse roll on top.
(c) Up vertical half-wave followed by curls on either side.
(d) Crown and nape hair falls in loose curls on the neck.

FIGURE 181. MIDDY HAIRCUT
in combination with—

(a) Top and sides are cut to reverse roll length.

DETAILS:
(a) Ear-to-ear part plus right side part.
(b) The left side hair has an up vertical half-wave, and combines with the top hair to produce the half-wave reverse roll on top.
(c) The right side hair is arranged in a high reverse roll.
(d) There are a few soft curls back of each ear.
(e) The nape hair swirls up and combines with the crown hair to produce a large flat roll in the crown area.

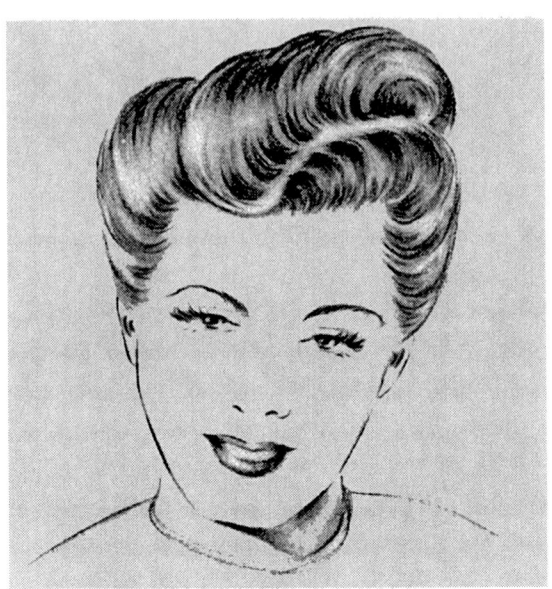

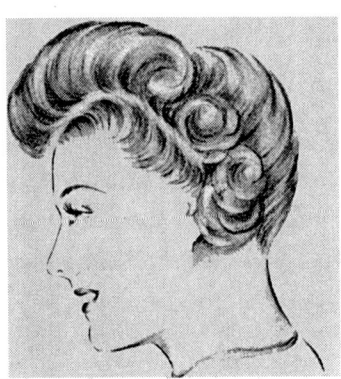

FIGURE 182. This is the left side view of the style shown in Figure 181.

FIGURE 183. MIDDY HAIRCUT
in combination with—

(a) Top hair is cut to full wave bangs length.
(b) Sides are full wave reverse roll length.

DETAILS:
(a) Ear-to-ear part plus "V" part.
(b) Full wave bangs.
(c) Full wave reverse roll at both sides.
(d) The crown and nape hair is combed down and arranged in a roll on the neck.

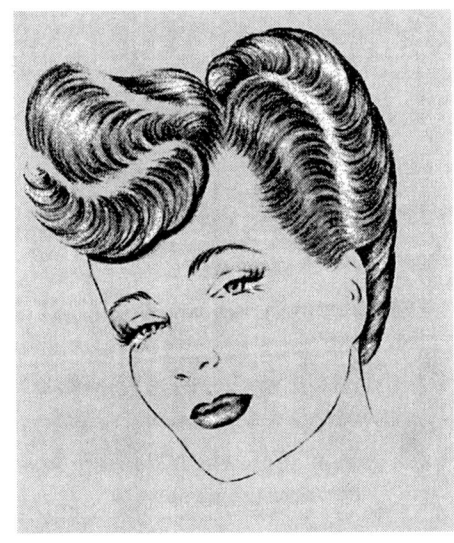

FIGURE 184. SHINGLE HAIRCUT

DETAILS:

(a) "V" part.

(b) Half-wave reverse roll on top.

(c) Both sides have an up vertical half-wave followed by soft curls.

(d) The crown and nape hair swirls to the left, and has shadow waves.

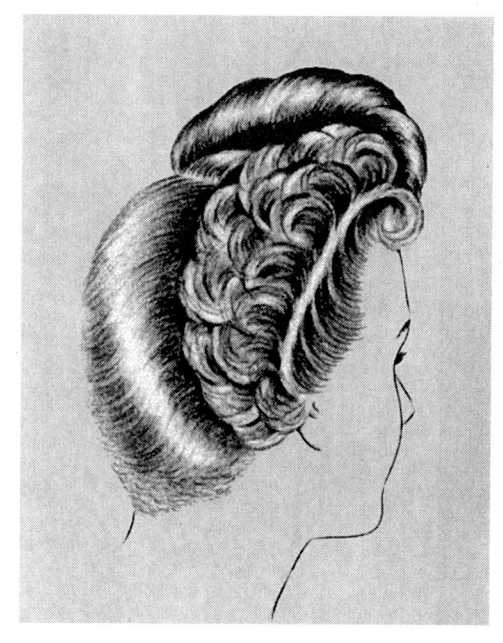

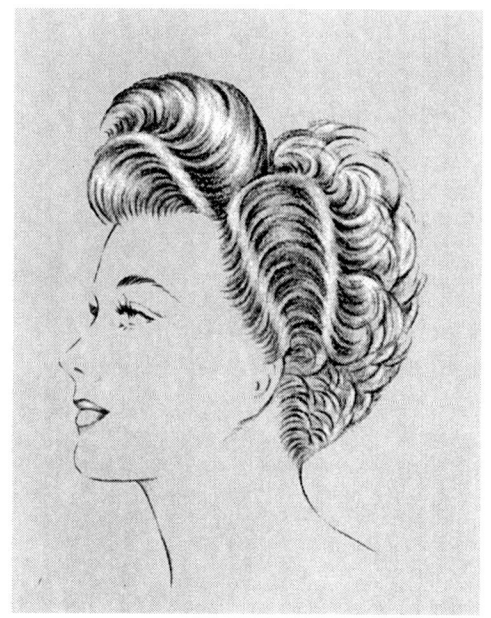

FIGURE 185.
SHINGLE PLUS HAIRCUT

DETAILS:

(a) Rectangular part.

(b) Half-wave reverse roll on top.

(c) Both sides have a wide vertical wave followed by curled ends that flare into place.

(d) The hair at the neck is brushed up and allowed to fall carelessly.

101

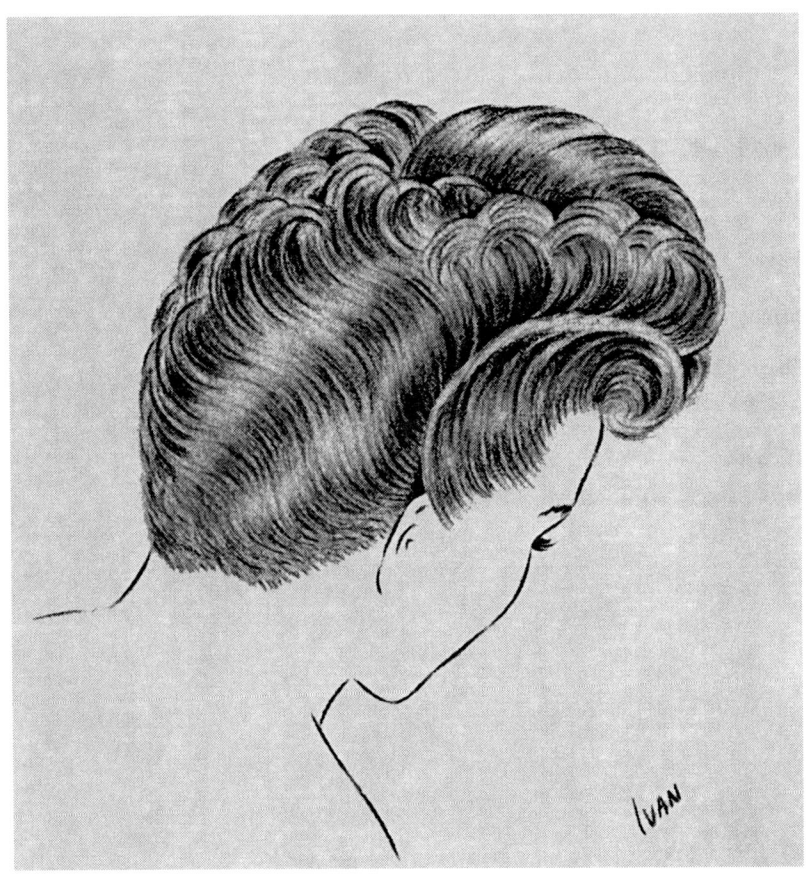

FIGURE 186. SHINGLE HAIRCUT
DETAILS:
- (a) "V" part.
- (b) Forward roll on top combines with fluff bangs.
- (c) Both sides have an up vertical half-wave followed by wispy curls.
- (d) Shadow-waved nape hair swirls up and flares.

THE HAIRSTYLE MUST BE SUITABLE TO THE OCCASION...

When designing hairstyles we must keep in mind the occasion on which they will be worn. The same common sense you use in selecting clothes that are suitable to the occasion applies equally well to the selection of the proper hairstyles. Wearing a tight-fitting formal while horseback riding would be just as ridiculous as selecting a high fashion coiffure to wear while swimming.

There are hundreds of occasions, and to discuss each of them individually would lead to confusion, so this subject will be broken down into these four categories: sports, business, semi-formal, and formal.

1. HAIRSTYLES FOR SPORTS

Sports hairstyles must first of all be simple and easily combed. Baby and Middy Haircuts may be worn in loose curls or fluff, while Middy Plus and Long Haircuts might require bobby pins, combs, ribbons, or snoods to control the hair.

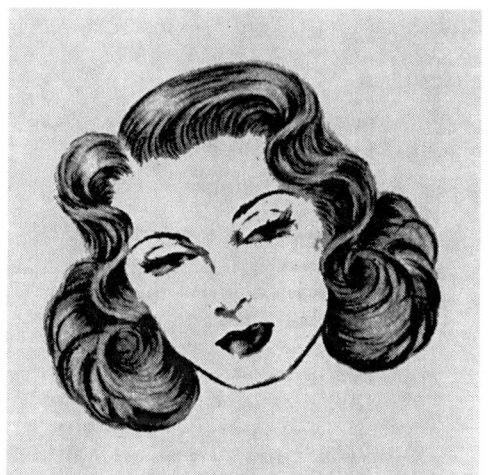

FIGURE 187. MIDDY PLUS HAIRCUT DETAILS:
   (a) Wide horizontal waves.
   (b) Large casual roll with loose ends showing.

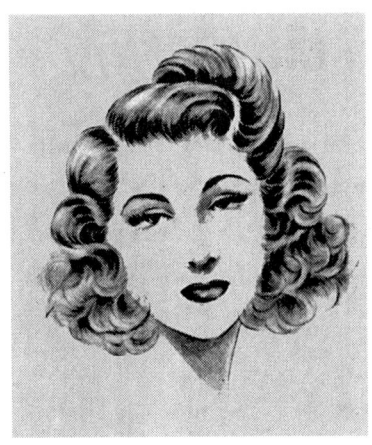

FIGURE 188. MIDDY PLUS HAIRCUT
in combination with—
(a) The top hair is cut to reverse roll length.

DETAILS:
(a) The rectangular part includes the left side hair from the temple up.
(b) Modified half-wave reverse roll.
(c) The left side has a diagonal half-wave followed by soft curls.
(d) The right side has a complete horizontal wave with soft curls.
(e) The back is smooth with loose curls on the neck.

REMARKS:
(a) Observe the model's heart-shaped face and how the fullness of the hair at the sides rounds out her pointed chin.

FIGURE 189. MIDDY PLUS HAIRCUT
DETAILS:
(a) Rectangular part.
(b) Top hair is arranged in a combination of fluff bangs and a modified stand-up half-wave.
(c) Diagonal half-wave over each ear.
(d) Fluff over the ears and on the neck.

REMARKS:
(a) Since this style, featuring the diagonal half-wave over the ears, is so popular and difficult to do, setting instructions are given below.

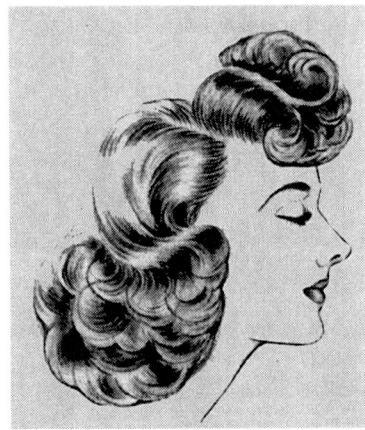

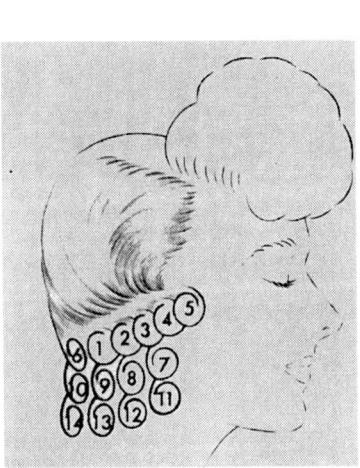

FIGURE 190. INSTRUCTIONS FOR SETTING A DIAGONAL HALF-WAVE OVER THE EARS.

These are the three tricks used in setting beautiful, diagonal half-waves over the ears:
(a) The hair at the temples is combed back away from the face.
(b) Crown and nape hair is "borrowed" and combed forward to help make the diagonal half-wave over the ear. *Be sure the half-wave slants up.*
(c) Curls numbered "1" through "5" take a backward direction. The others shown in this illustration turn forward. Setting these curls in opposite directions produces additional fullness over the ears after the hair is combed out.

2. HAIRSTYLES FOR BUSINESS

The last advice a business school gives to the graduating student is, "When you are to be interviewed for a new job, be sure your clothes are smart and your hairdress is neat." There can be no doubt about it, the hairdress does suggest the business efficiency of the wearer. If her hair is long, stringy, and poorly shaped, she will immediately be sized up as a sloppy, indifferent, careless worker. On the other hand, a neat, smoothly coiffed applicant instantly gives her prospective employer the impression that her work will be accurate and that she will be an asset to the business.

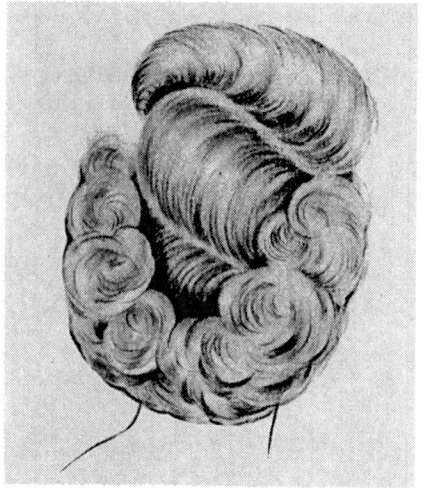

FIGURE 191. MIDDY HAIRCUT
in combination with—

(a) The nape and crown hair above the back diagonal part is about six inches in length.
(b) The top hair is full wave bangs length.

DETAILS:
(a) Back diagonal part plus two side parts.
(b) The bangs have one complete wave.
(c) The sides have an up vertical half-wave followed by curls.

FIGURE 192. LONG HAIRCUT
in combination with—

(a) Top and sides are reverse roll length.

DETAILS:
(a) Ear-to-ear part.
(b) Continuous roll all around the head.

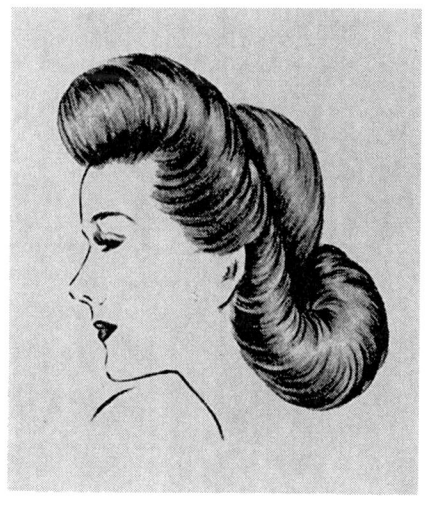

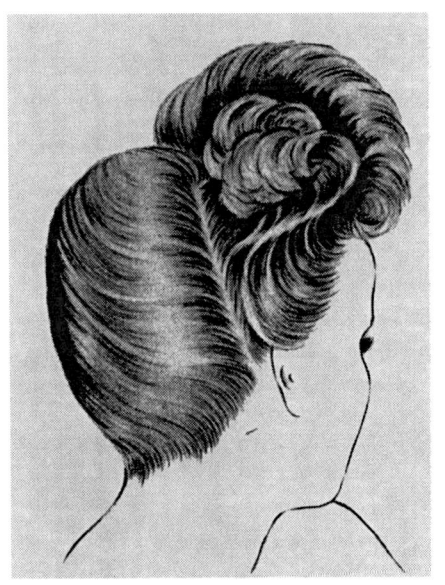

FIGURE 193. LONG HAIRCUT
in combination with—

(a) Top hair is cut to forward roll bangs length.

DETAILS:
(a) Modified ear-to-ear part.
(b) Half-wave bangs.
(c) Both left and right sides have an up diagonal half-wave followed by curls.
(d) The nape and crown hair swirls up and is folded into a flat roll on the left side of the head.

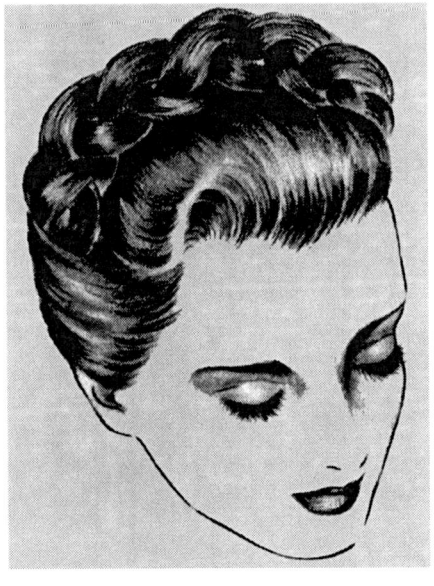

FIGURE 194. SHINGLE HAIRCUT

DETAILS:
(a) An extra wide rectangular part.
(b) The top hair goes almost straight back, but has a short half-wave above the right eye.
(c) Both sides are combed over, and tucked under the ends of the braided hair-piece.
(d) The crown and nape hair is swirled and has two large shadow waves.

REMARKS:
(a) If the hair is long enough, this style may be duplicated without the use of the braided hair-piece.
(b) This coronet style is recommended for the more sophisticated business executive.

3. SEMI-FORMAL HAIRSTYLES

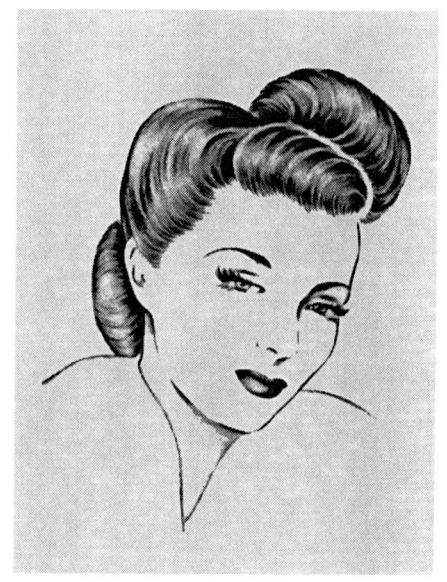

FIGURE 195. LONG HAIRCUT
in combination with—

(a) Top and sides are cut to half-wave reverse roll length.

DETAILS:
(a) Ear-to-ear part plus two side parts.
(b) Stand-up half-wave reverse roll on top.
(c) Sides are swept up, and the ends tucked under the roll.
(d) Crown and nape hair is combed down and fashioned over a chignon frame or rat.

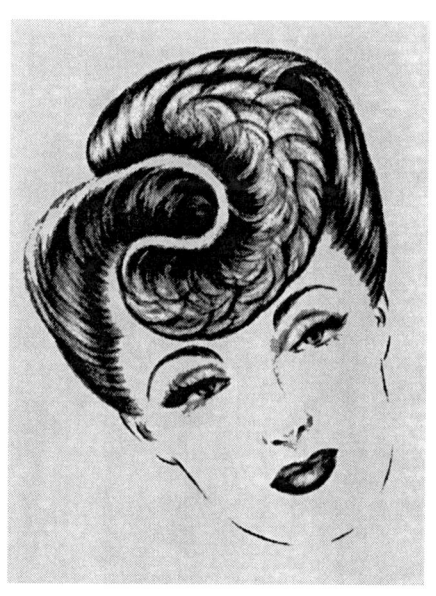

FIGURE 196. MIDDY HAIRCUT
in combination with—

(a) Sides are reverse roll length.

DETAILS:
(a) Ear-to-ear part plus up diagonal left side part.
(b) Left side hair is swept up into a high forward roll.
(c) Right side hair is combed up and fashioned into modified French bangs.
(d) The crown and nape hair is gathered into a cluster of curls on the center of the neck.

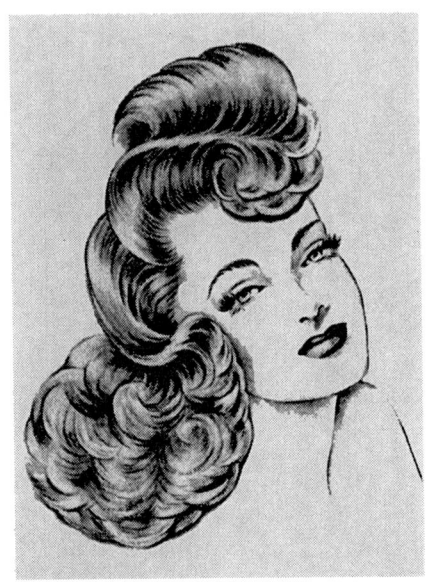

FIGURE 197. LONG HAIRCUT
in combination with—
(a) Top hair is cut to half-wave pomp length.
(b) Fringe bangs are cut two inches in length.

DETAILS:
(a) The part extends from temple to temple.
(b) Combination of half-wave pomp and fringe bangs.
(c) Diagonal half-wave over each ear.
(d) Fluff at neck and over ears.

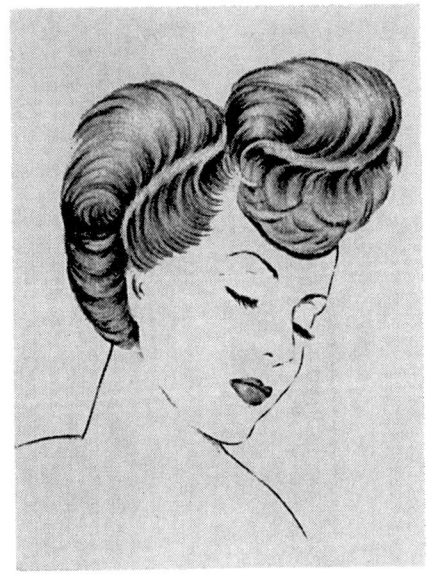

FIGURE 198. MIDDY HAIRCUT
in combination with—
(a) Top hair is cut to half-wave bangs length.
(b) Sides are half-wave reverse roll length.

DETAILS:
(a) "V" part plus center back part.
(b) Half-wave bangs.
(c) Up vertical half-wave reverse roll at the sides.
(d) Forward roll back of each ear.

4. FORMAL HAIRSTYLES

Formal, lacquered coiffures without a hair out of place suggest sophistication, wealth, and high fashion. Notice that the expensive fur, rare jewel, and fine automobile advertisements in Vogue and Harper's Bazaar usually show a beautiful, formally-coiffed model to accent the product being advertised. This is not an accident. The advertisers know only too well that a high fashion hairstyle will automatically suggest to the reader that the model is a woman of refinement and is financially able to own that expensive automobile or ermine herself.

When that long looked-forward-to-prom, annual company formal, or the special celebration at Ciro's or the Stork Club finally arrives, your patrons will want you to "shoot the works" and put their hair up. Their jeweled ear-tips, orchids or hair ornaments will compliment your up-coiffure creations. *But don't forget*—a formal hairdress is not all-important in itself. *If a hairdress is not flattering, it is a failure!*

We have all seen formal hairdresses that were a work of art and would have been out of this world IF Lana Turner or Hedy Lamarr had worn them, but on Mabel McGillicuddy they looked like—well, you know what I mean. For this reason, it may be advisable to try your creation at least once before the formal, and make changes if necessary.

General suggestions for designing formal coiffures:

    Avoid narrow waves and tight curls.

    Don't overload the hairdress with countless details.

    Keep the details large and soft-looking.

    Use shadow waves, and insert rats or tease the hair to make details appear soft and natural looking.

    Concentrate on up-lines.

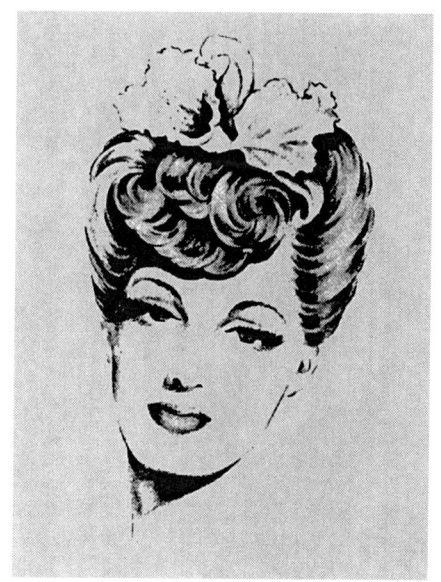

FIGURE 199. LONG HAIRCUT
    in combination with—

    (a) Sides are cut to reverse roll length.

DETAILS:

    (a) Ear-to-ear part plus two side parts.

    (b) Fluff bangs.

    (c) Reverse roll on both sides.

    (d) Nape and crown hair is swept up and placed in large flat rolls just back of the orchid.

REMARKS:

    (a) The orchid serves a double purpose—it lends a formal atmosphere, and gives needed height to the style.

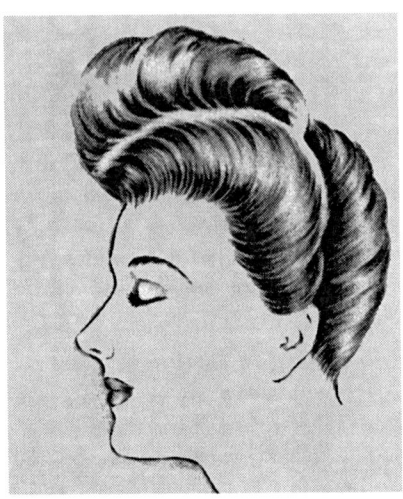

FIGURE 200. MIDDY PLUS HAIRCUT
in combination with—
 (a) Top and sides are reverse roll length.

DETAILS:
 (a) Ear-to-ear part plus right side part.
 (b) The left side hair is draped up to combine with the top hair in producing the modified half-wave reverse roll.
 (c) The right side hair is combed into a high reverse roll.
 (d) The nape and crown hair is folded into a large flat roll in the crown area.

FIGURE 201. LONG HAIRCUT
in combination with—
 (a) The sides are cut to reverse roll length.

DETAILS:
 (a) Rectangular part.
 (b) Stand-up half-wave followed by curls.
 (c) The right and left side hair combines with the nape and crown hair to produce a large flat roll just back of the curls.

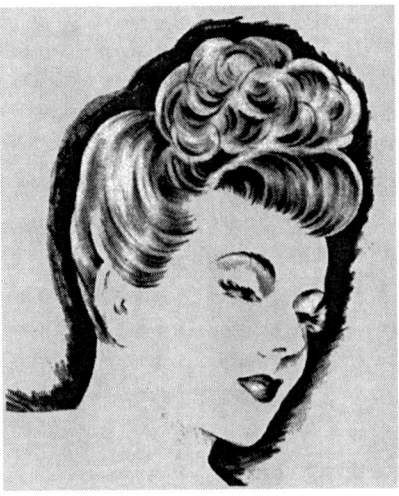

FIGURE 202. LONG HAIRCUT
in combination with—
 (a) The fluff bangs are three inches in length.
 (b) Top and sides are cut to reverse roll length.

DETAILS:
 (a) Back diagonal part plus rectangular part.
 (b) Fluff bangs above right eye.
 (c) Top half-wave reverse roll.
 (d) The remaining hair is folded in two flat rolls on either side of the back diagonal part.

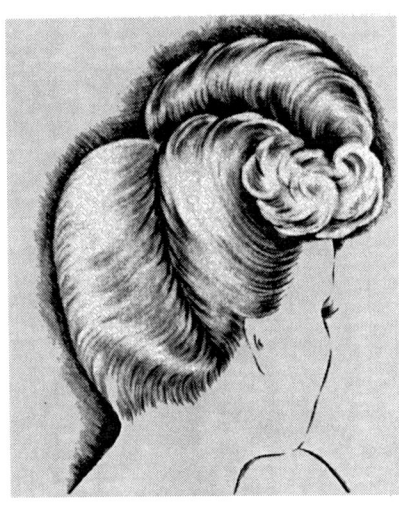

Conclusion . . .

It is my sincere desire that this Volume will, in some measure,

contribute to the art of Hairshaping and Hairstyling

IVAN

ACKNOWLEDGMENTS

MY MOTHER, for her advice and encouragement

FREDERICK L. RICHARDS, for his photography

ROBERT W. BOONE, for his design of this Volume

PERC WESTMORE, for his professional advice

HELEN HUNT, for her professional advice

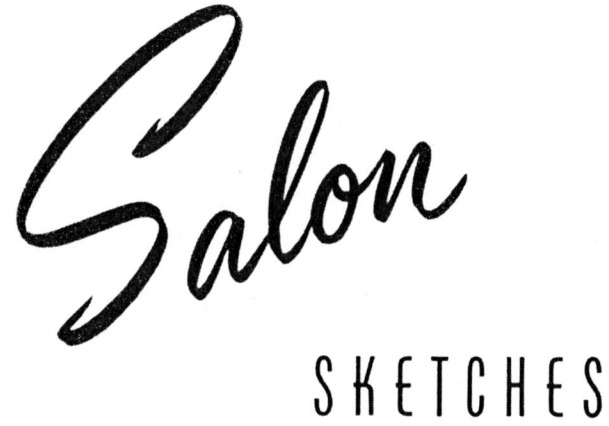

Salon
SKETCHES

The remaining sketches, illustrating formal and high fashion coiffures, are reproduced full page size so you may cut them out and frame them for window and booth advertising in your Salon.

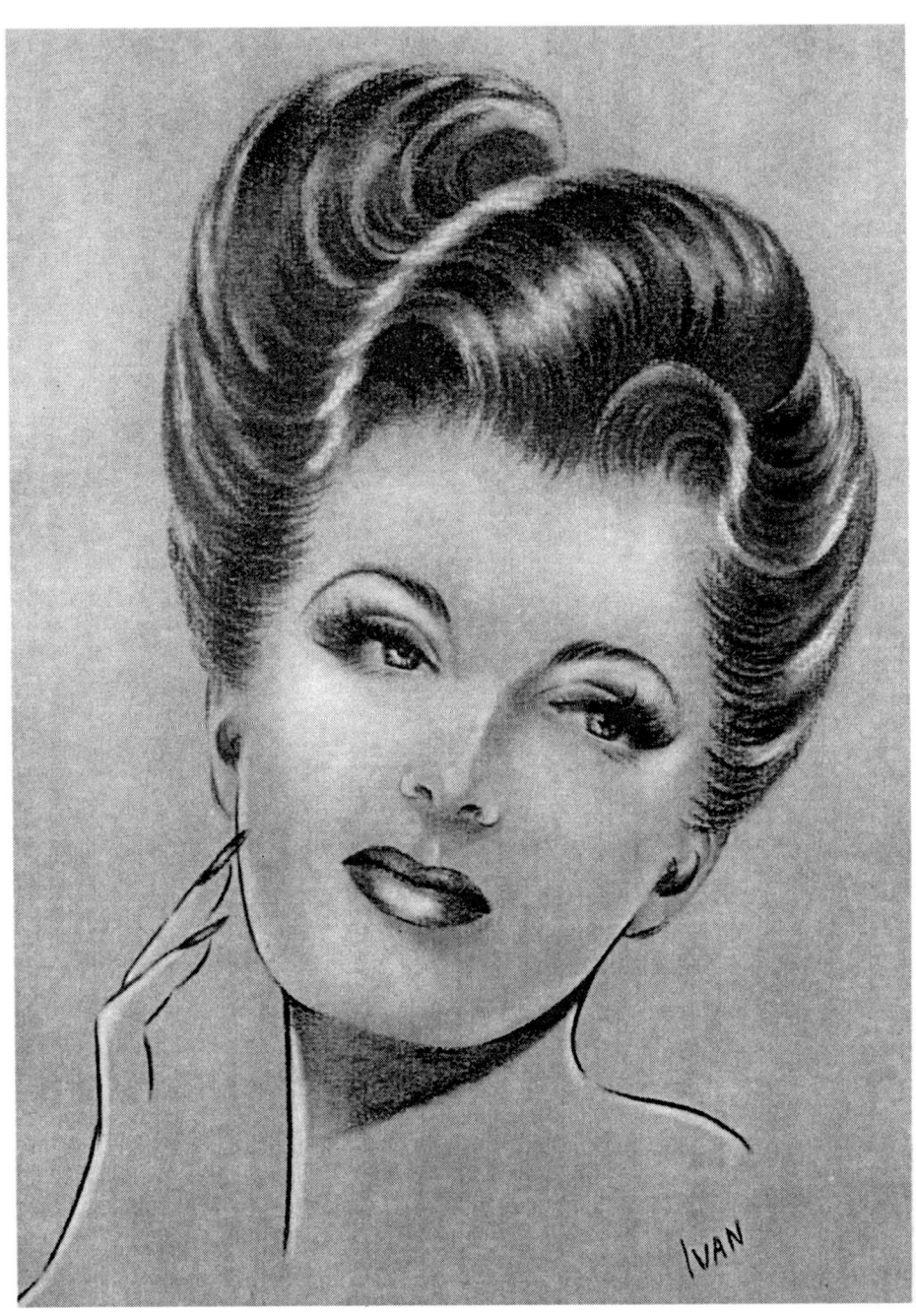

FIGURE 203

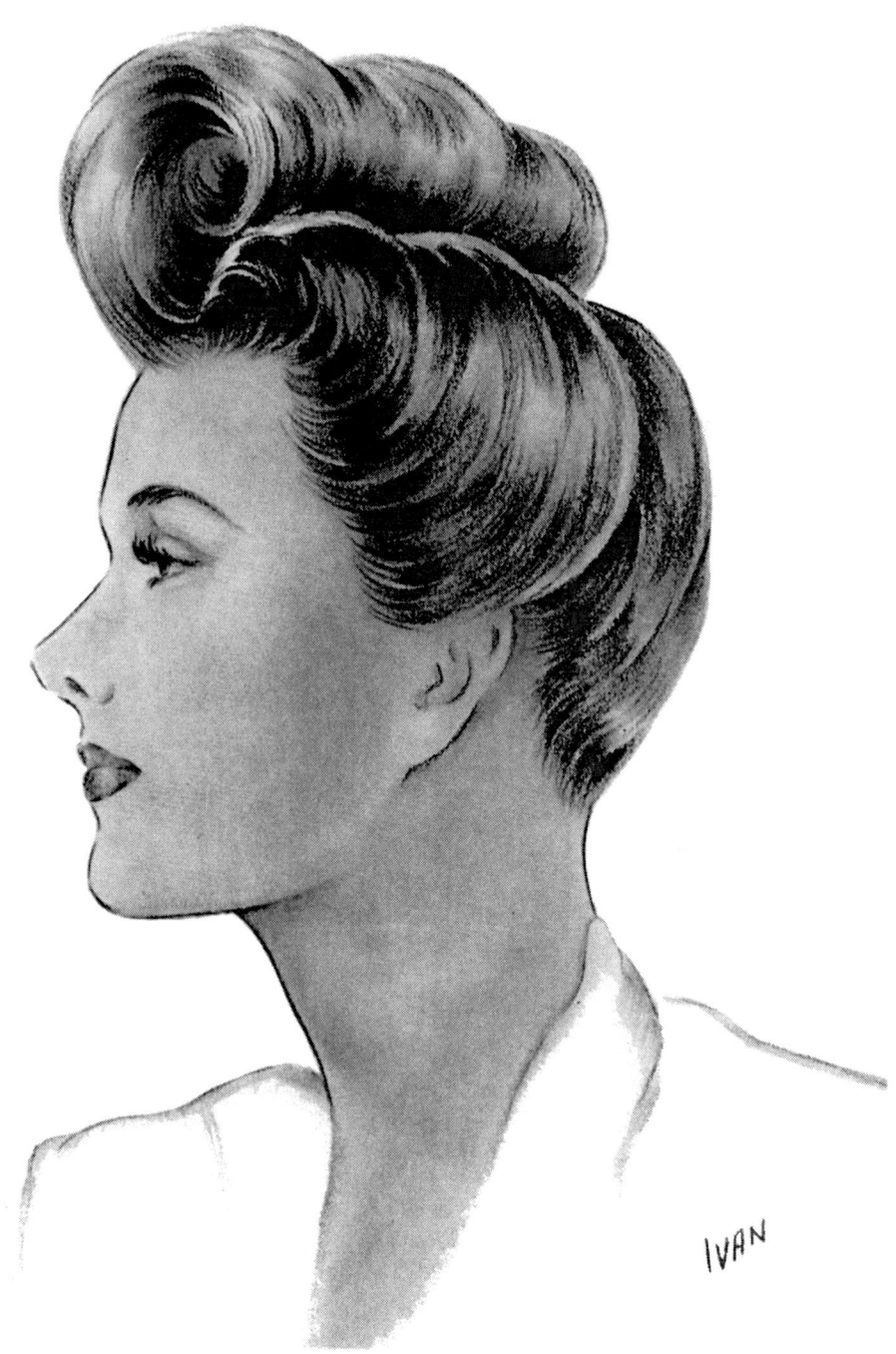

FIGURE 204

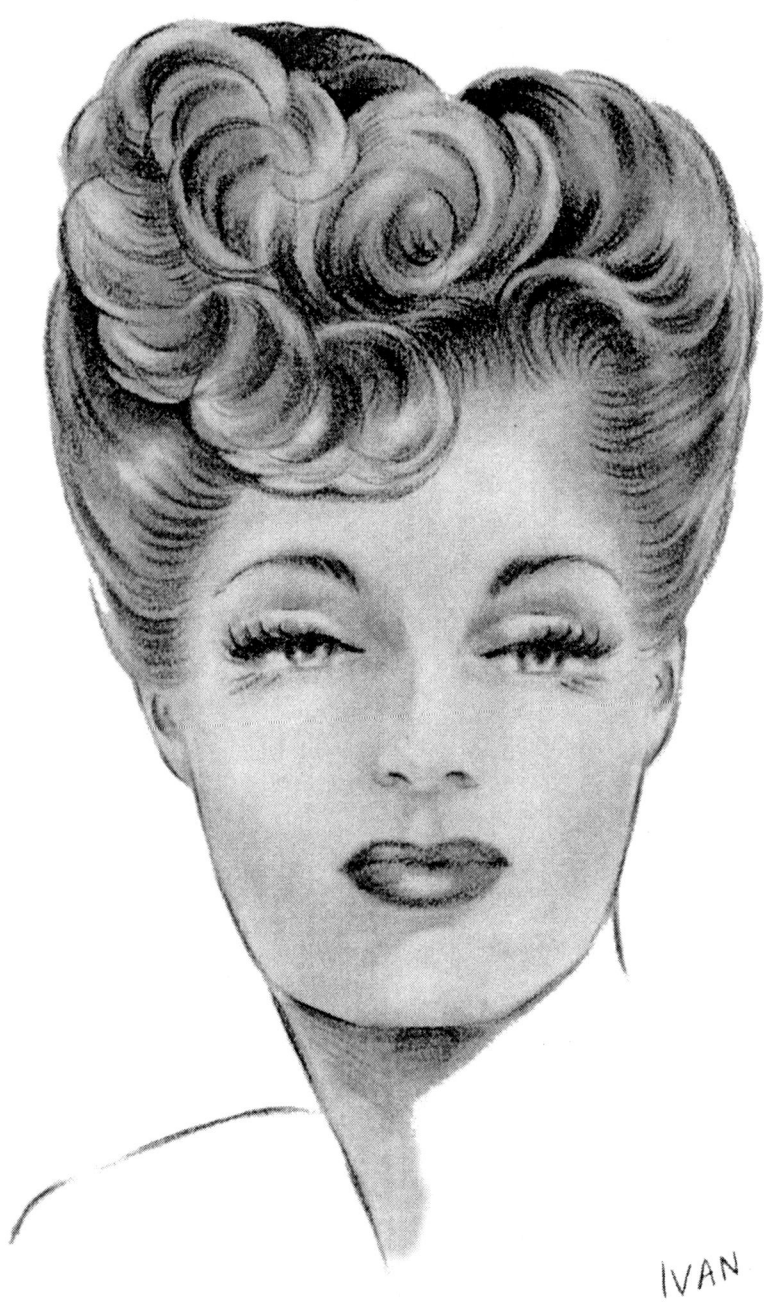

FIGURE 205

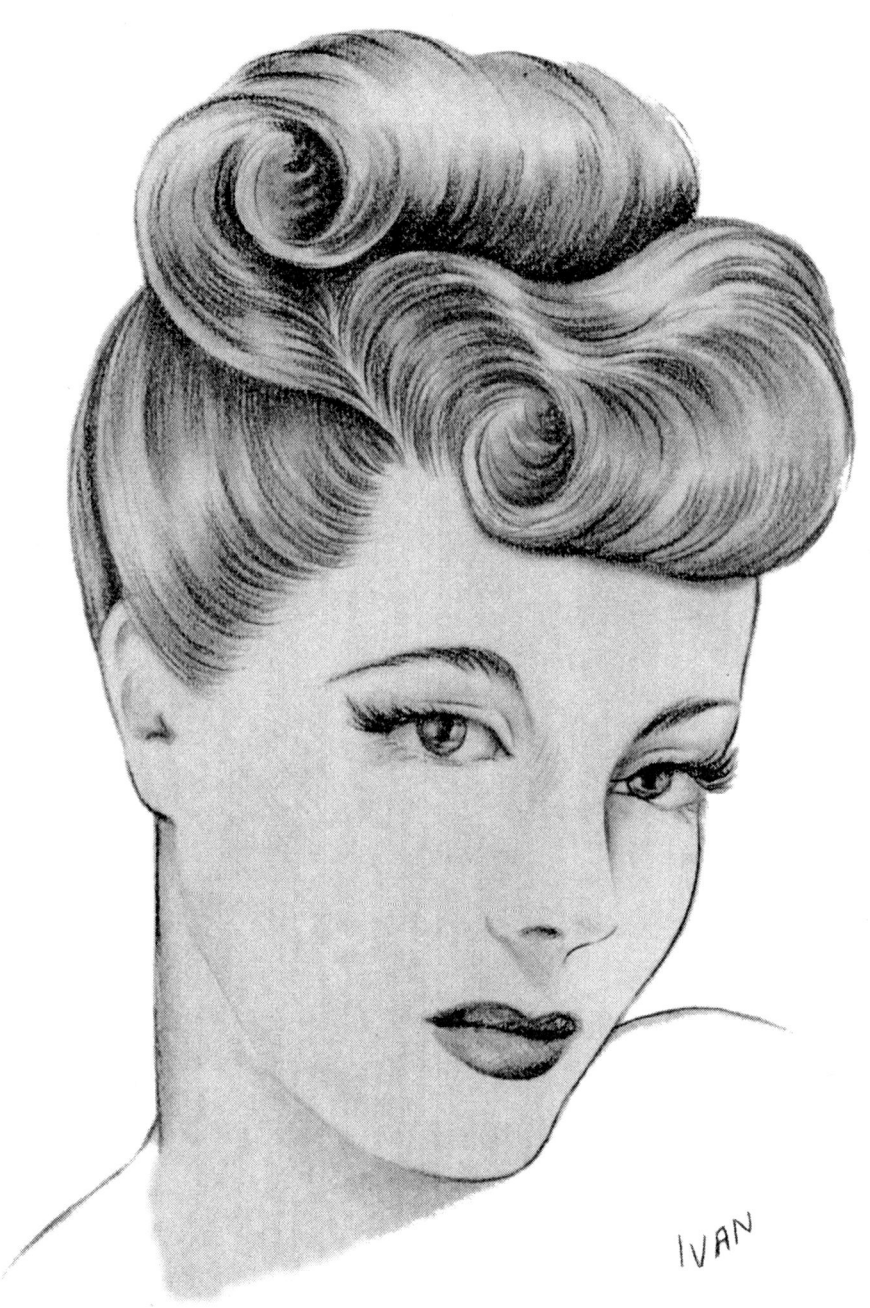

FIGURE 206

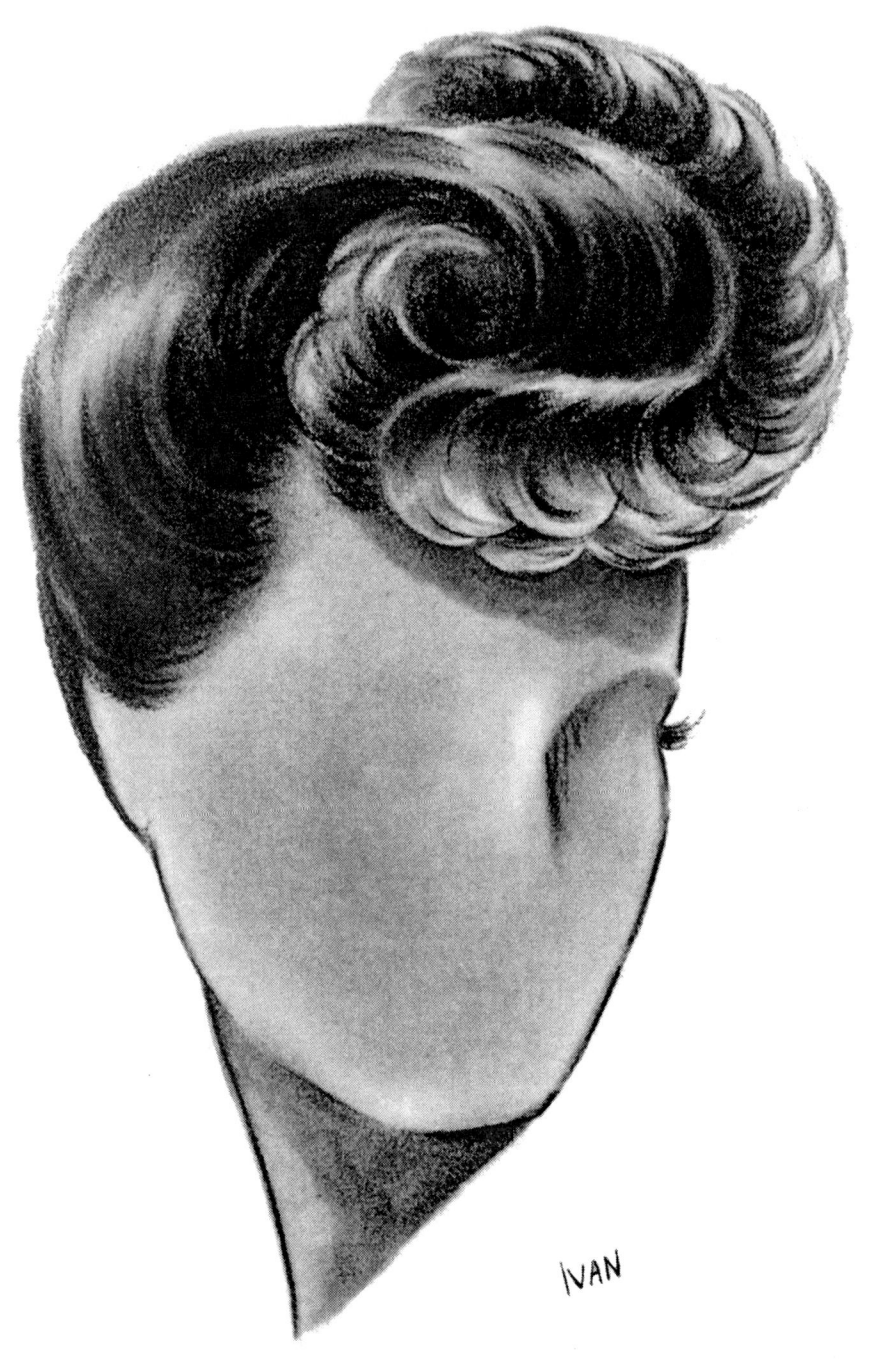

FIGURE 207

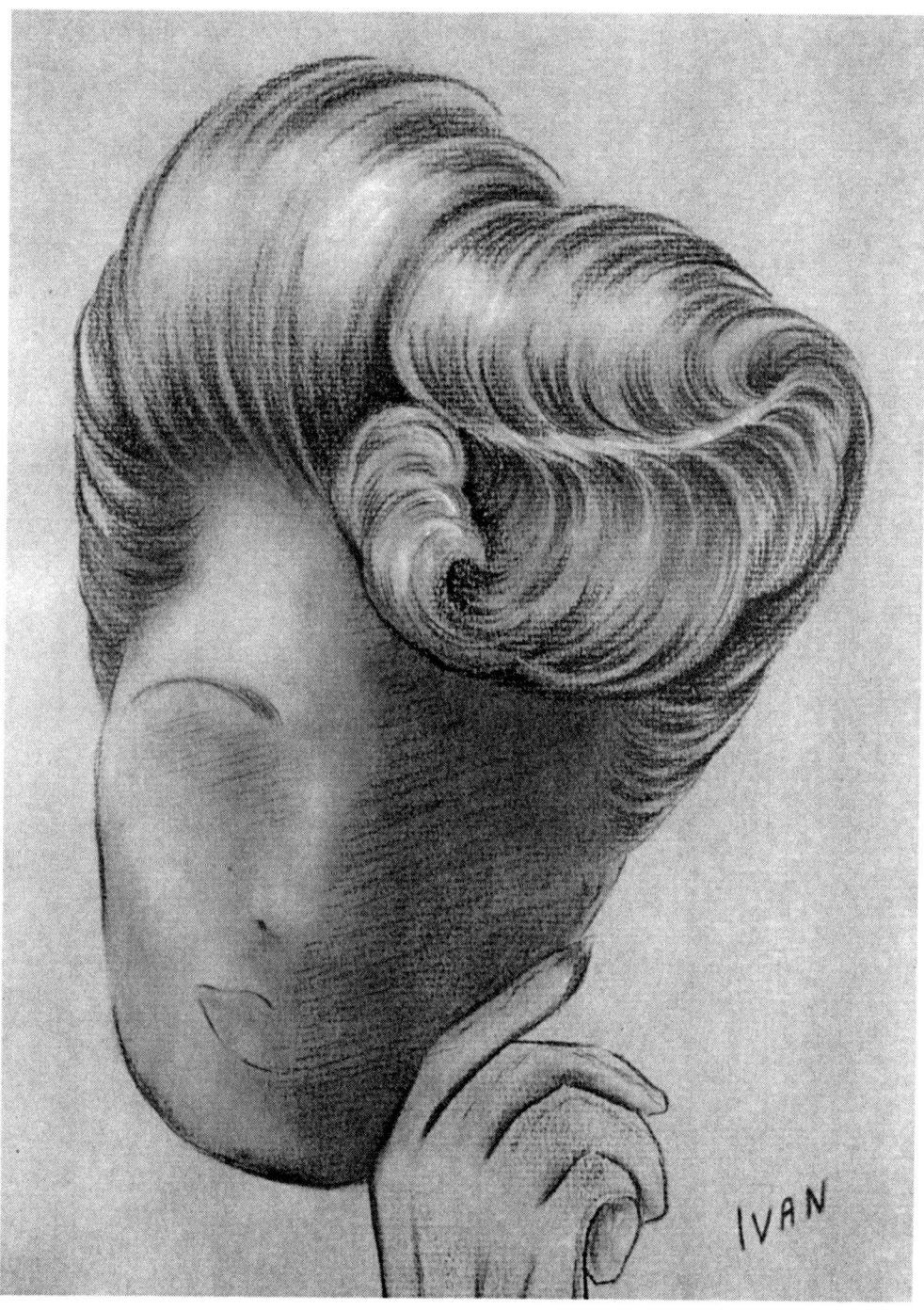

FIGURE 208

Printed in the United States
220823BV00004B/1/P